George N. Touliatos, MD

BODYBUILDING:
THE GOOD, THE BAD &
THE UGLY

Copyrights ® 2018. George N.Touliatos, MD

Editing by Dimos Velenjas

Book design by: Selfpublishing Onlinewww.selfpublishingonline.eu

August 2018

Books are not transferable. All Rights Are Reserved. No part of this book may be used or reproduced in any manner without written permission, except in the case of brief quotations embodied in critical articles and reviews. The unauthorized reproduction or distribution of this copyrighted work Is illegal. No part of this book may be scanned, uploaded or distributed via the Internet or any other means, electronic

ISBN: 9781718065482

The Hippocratic Oath

I swear by Apollo the Healer, by Asclepius, by Hygeia, by Panacea, and by all the gods and goddesses, making them my witnesses, that I will carry out, according to my ability and judgment, this oath and this indenture.

To hold my teacher in this art equal to my own parents; to make him partner in my livelihood; when he is in need of money to share mine with him; to consider his family as my own brothers, and to teach them this art, if they want to learn it, without fee or indenture; to impart precept, oral instruction, and all other instruction to my own sons, the sons of my teacher, and to indentured pupils who have taken the physician's oath, but to nobody else.

I will use treatment to help the sick according to my ability and judgment, but never with a view to injury and wrong-doing. Neither will I administer a poison to anybody when asked to do so, nor will I suggest such a course. Similarly I will not give to a woman a pessary to cause abortion. But I will keep pure and holy both my life and my art. I will not use the knife, not even, verily, on sufferers from stone, but I will give place to such as are craftsmen therein.

Into whatsoever houses I enter, I will enter to help the sick, and I will abstain from all intentional wrong-doing and harm, especially from abusing the bodies of man or woman, bond or free. And whatsoever I shall see or hear in the course of my profession, as well as outside my profession in my intercourse with men, if it be what should not be published abroad, I will never divulge, holding such things to be holy secrets.

Now if I carry out this oath, and break it not, may I gain for ever reputation among all men for my life and for my art; but if I transgress it and forswear myself, may the opposite befall me.

Acknowledgements

I would like to thank a few people, whose contribution was valuable.

-Nelson Vergel, the author of "Testosterone: A man's guide" and creator of www.excelmale.com. His contribution to the English translation of my latest book was a major achievement without any doubt. We exchanged priceless scientific information online and I am thankful for that interaction.

-Dr.Thomas O'Connor,the anabolic Doc in USA,medical associate of Anabolics 11th edition book,columnist of Muscular Development magazine and author of the book "America on steroids,a time to heal". Dr.O is a pioneer in what he does and I am greatful to his belief and trust in my work.

-Dr.John Crisler, the author of "TRT". Brilliant physician with vast experience in AAS and TRT use in men. Thank you for your kindness.

-Dr.Massimo Spattini, the author of "Com diet and spot reduction". Fortuned to be tutored by him personally, he is still a role model, as we serve the same passion for bodybuilding.

-Dr.Rand Mc Clain for giving me a tremendous opportunity to be hosted in his show on Jay Cutler TV

-Jay Cambell, author of "TRT manual" and creator of www.trtrevolution.com. Wise open minded fellow, who gave me the opportunity to talk in his podcast.

-Rick Collins, theworld's finest expert regarding thesteroid law. I had the privilege of meeting him, exchanging valuable ideas about the iron sport and PED's use.

-Carl Lanore, creator of Super Human Radio.A sharp mind who invited me five times in his live show. Glad to have met Carl and Alisa in Columbus, OH.

-Patrick Arnold, the mastermind chemist.A legendary scientist who has developed extensive research on Keto supplements.

Meeting him was quite an experience, as well as interacting online. Thank you for your time sir.

-Frank Sepe, my inspiration during my early days of fitness. Hopefully I met him almost two decades later, at the Arnold's festival. His vast experience is something you rarely found.

-Jay Cutler, 4x times Mr. Olympia. I was thrilled each time we met. We had the chance of having two seminars held in Greece and to meet twice, in ASC and FIBO EXPOs 2016.Spending time with him was a dream of a life time. Champ, keep motivating us.

-Milos Sarcev, the best ambassador of professional bodybuilding in Balkans.Had the pleasure of meeting him in Athens and promised him one day i will mail him my English book.Cant thank him enough for his promotion online.

-Dave Palumbo, the anabolic freak of MD magazine.He believed in my potential and gave me the opportunity to have be intervied twice, on line in his RXMUSCLE channel.One of the most knowledgable and well known people in the sport,worldwide.

-Ron Harris, for his acknowledgment and the opportunities he gave me in Muscular Development TV.

-Steve Blechman, editor in chief of Muscular Development magazine in USA. This was an opportunity of a life time and a dream that came true. Four years ago I was a medical contributor in the Greek translated edition and now the time has finally arrived for my international carrier overseas. Its such an honor that we met in Las Vegas.

-

-William Lleweyn, last but not least, Creator of www.roidtest.com, www.anabolic.org, CEO of Molecular Nutrition, author of Anabolics books. He is the man who believed in my potential and accomplished my dream: expanding my knowledge, far from domestic borders.

Truly, I would never thought of becoming international five years ago, when I published my first book. To him I owe my international carrier. I am very grateful to him and his associate, Tim Zakowski. Proud to be a member of his latest masterpiece, Anabolics book 11th edition. Glad that we finaly met in Denver.

This book is dedicated to those who believed in me and my vision:

My family mostly and my followers.

RECOMMENDATIONS

"Dr.George Touliatos,is one of our leading contributors at www.anabolic.org.

His blend of first hand bodybuilding experience,along with his impressive academic and professional backgrounds,makes him one of the world's foremost experts on performance enhancing drugs".

William Llewellyn

Creator of Roidtest.com, Anabolic.org

CEO of Molecular Nutrition, author of Anabolics books.

"Dr.Touliatos is one of the very few true experts on Anabolic Steroids and health consequences in the world".

Thomas O'Connor, MD

Clinical instructor of medicine, Department of Medicine, University of Connenticut School of Medicine, Anabolics book 2017 Medical Contributor.

Collumnist of Muscular Development magazine

"Nice compilation of everything, well organised".

Dave Palumbo

NPC superheavy weight first runner up,

Anabolic freak, Muscular Development magazine,

Creator of RXmuscle.com

"A fascinating book by George Touliatos MD, from the unique perspective of a physician with firsthand knowledge of anabolic steroids for bodybuilding".

Rick Collins

Attorney at law of bodybuilding community

Authror of Legal Muscle book

Collumnist at Muscular Development magazine

"Dr Touliatos wrote this enlightening book not only from the point of view of a physician but also from a ex-user of performance enhancing drugs. He reviews many products currently used by athletes and bodybuilders to help people exploring their use to learn about the benefits and potential side effects of each one. Highly recommended for people who want to learn PED information beyond what they find online".

Nelson Vergel, author of "Testosterone,a man's guide"

Creator of excelmale.com

"I like your book, you're a very smart dude "

John Romano

Former Muscular Development columnist

T-Nation columnist

Bigger, stronger, faster documentary

TABLE OF CONTENTS

EVOLUTION OF PEDS 4
DOPING-ANTIDOPING STRATEGIES 8
HOW ATHLETES GET DOPED 13
PEDS IN MODERN SOCIETY 18
THE SIGNIFICANCE OF MEDICAL PREVENTION IN BODYBUILDING 22
CNS STIMULANTS 26

    CLENBUTEROL HYDROCHLORIDE (Clenbuterol HCL) 26
    EPHEDRINE HYDROCHLORIDE (Ephedrine HCL) 28
    YOHIMBINE HYDROCHLORIDE 30
    CAFFEINE 31
    THYROXINE T4 (Thyroxine) 33
    AMPHETAMINES 34

ANABOLIC HORMONES 36

    SOMATROPIN – GROWTH HORMONE (HGH) 36
    HGH GUT 42
    PEPTIDES (Secretagogues) 46
    INSULIN AND SOMATOMEDIN C (Insulin & IGF-1) 48
    TESTOSTERONE 52

TESTOSTERONE'S SYNTHETIC DERIVATIVES 62

    17 ALKYLATED AAS 62
    OTHER AAS 70

PHARMAKOKINETICS OF AAS 78

AUTHENTICITY OF AAS 81

    INTRAMUSCULAR ABSCESS 83
    ERYTHROPOIESIS AND ATHLETIC PERFORMANCE 89
    CORTICOSTEROIDS 91
    STEROID LETHARGY EFFECT 93
    DIURETICS 95
    AROMATASE INHIBITORS 98
    ARTHRALGIA OF AROMATASE INHIBITORS 100
    AROMATASE INHIBITORS AND VISUAL DISORDERS 103
    ESTROGEN FACTS 105
    GYNECOMASTIA 107
    SELECTIVE ANDROGEN RECEPTOR MODULATORS 109
    MEDICAL INDICATIONSFOR THERAPEUTIC ADMINISTRATIONOF PEDs 111

POST CYCLE THERAPY (PCT) 114
HORMONAL REPLACEMENT THERAPY (HRT) AS A RESULT OF ANDROGEN INDUCED HYPOGONADISM (AIH-AAS ABUSE) 117
SUPPRESSION OF THE PITUITARY-HYPOTHALAMIC-TESTICULAR AXIS, AS A RESULT OF AAS ABUSE 125

INDICATIVE AAS CYCLES 129

INDICATIVE CYCLE FOR BULKING 129
INDICATIVE CYCLE FOR CUTTING 132
LABORATORY TESTS – MONITORING THE PROFIL OF THE ATHLETE 136
    LABORATORY ASSESSMENT DURING PHYSICAL STRESS *139*
MAIN ADVERSEEFFECTS OF AAS 141
    1. CARDIOVASCULAR SYSTEM: *141*
    2. LIVER-BILIARY TRACT: *142*
    3. URINARY SYSTEM (KIDNEYS): *145*
    4. REPRODUCTIVE SYSTEM (SEX GLANDS) *146*
    5. HEMATOPOIETIC AND HAEMOSTATIC SYSTEM: *147*
    6. NEUROLOGICAL - PSYCHIATRIC: *147*
    7. IMMUNE SYSTEM: *148*
    8. CARCINOGENESIS: *148*
MAIN ADVERSE EFFECTS OF NON-AAS PEDs 149
    1) HGH (GROWTH HORMONE-SOMATROPIN): *149*
    2) INSULIN: *149*
    3) DIURETICS: *150*
    4) STIMULANTS: *150*
    5) Recombinant human erythropoietin (-rEPO) *153*

MECHANISMS OF DAMAGE BY PEDS USE 154

CARDIOVASCULAR SYSTEM 154
    AAS - INDUCED HYPERTENSION *157*
    AAS AND HOMOCYSTEINE *160*
GENITOURINARY SYSTEM 163
HEMATOPOIETIC SYSTEM 166
    MUSCLE GROWTH AND CANCER *169*

PREVENTION OF SIDE-EFFECTS OF PEDS USE 170

LIFESTYLE PREVENTIVE TIPS ALONG WITH PEDS USE 170
HOW PRO'S CYCLE AAS 172
EXERCISE INDUCED CARDIAC REMODELING 174
THE IMPORTANCE OF EXERCISE IN COMPARISON TO STATINES, REGARDING PREVENTION AND TREATMENT OF CARDIOVASCULAR EPISODES 177
ANDROGEN EMOTIONAL TOXICITY SYNDROME 179
PREPARING FOR A SHOW 184
POSSING 190

EPILOGUE 193

WHAT BODYBUILDING IS ALL ABOUT? 193

BODYBUILDING AND MORTALITY	197
TOP 100 BODYBUILDERS OF ALL TIME	200

SELF CRITISISM 205

REFERENCES 207

INTERVIEW 212

CV

PICTURES

PREFACE

Health is the most important gift of all, because only if we are healthy we are able to achieve our accomplishments.

As a doctor, I do know that medical prevention, through proper life style, or medical examinations, provide longevity. However, during my medical carrier I realised that, there are unknown pathogenesis of certain diseases. Quality of living in third age ensures a decent living when the individual can take care of himself, especially if he is independent on that. If we were able to realise our bad living habits would cost us in the far future, I am positive we would have stopped them. Everybody seems to regret that during suffering, when is seriously ill.

Health is an expensive gift nowadays in the modern world. In case you can't afford getting hospitalised, your chances are poor to survive. It is better some patients to pass out shortly, rather than being a torture for themselves and their relatives as well. During my athletic carrier, I realised that being out of injuries, or any other kind of medical condition, I was able to achieve my expectations.

I wish all doctors of the world were useless. However, the modern human spends tremendous time of energy and time in order to make money and afterwards spends his fortune in order to improve his bad shape. Hippocrates, the father of modern medicine said, whatever is not cured by medication, is treated by scalpel; while Apostle Paul mentioned the importance of consulting a physician. I am deeply sorry to hear that my colleagues are getting profit in financial terms from the pain of their patients.

As a doctor I am against euthanasia. I do strongly believe that life is the most valuable gift on this earth and we have to live it till the end. Besides as a Christian I am against of it, even when the patient asks of it with despair. It is well known the case of "doctor death", Dr.Kevorkian in the United States. He terminated the life of more than hundred patients who asked for and fulfilled the terms for it. Eventually, he was convicted and spent over five years in jail for his "legal" crimes. Health in ancient Sparta and in the third Reich of Germany, were valuable gifts. As known, weak boys were thrown away as soon as they were born, while sick children were assassinated in gas chambers.

I wish they were no diseases in this world; but through fighting those diseases, modern medicine becomes stronger and more effective in order to provide longevity and class to our living.

Personal note

The title of this book, "the good, the bad & the ugly", briefly explains the deeper aspect of what iron sport is about and represents.

The good refers to the flashy and glamorous side of it. Tanned, oiled, shaved, ripped, veiny and muscular bodies posing on stage. Supreme physiques that reveal this majestic-but misunderstood sport.

The bad, encloses all the sacrifices as part of this discipline life style. Dedication, devotion, tunnel vision that basically build a strong character and will power.

The ugly side of bodybuilding is hardly revealed, simply because truth hurts and shocks.

Drug abuse leads to a plethora of side effects and diseases, making bodybuilding a potentially dangerous life style. Only a physician who walked his talk (as a former competitive bodybuilder), could say it better than anyone else, with reality.

EVOLUTION OF PEDS

Since the ancient time, humans had developed a competitive spirit in them, in order to be better against each others. The Olympic spirit with its motto: "Ciltius, Altius, fortius" meaning "faster, higher, stronger" included the terms of fair play in games. During the Olympic Games held in ancient Olympia, wrestlers of Pangration sport used to eat bull testicles to increase their power, through testosterone. During the first modern Olympics games in Athens, at 1896, performance enhancing methods took their initial steps. A cyclist was allegedly to have used the pain killer narcotic "strychnine", in order to avoid the feeling of pain and prolong his stamina.

In 1935 the Germans isolated testosterone in lab and manufactured in synthetic form (Nobel Prize, Chemistry 1939). Later, during World War II (WW2), the third Reich soldiers extensively abused injectable testosterone to sustain injuries and malnutrition, while aggressiveness and stamina were the major drawbacks.

Right after the end of the WW2 period, doping made its appearance in football and more specifically in the 1954 World Cup, held in Switzerland. West Germany was rumored of doping, almost half of the team that won the final against Hungary. Surprisingly, at half time score was 0-2 for the team of French Puskas. At the same year, American scientist Dr. John

Ziegler originally developed the most widespread anabolic steroid, methandrostenolone (Dianabol).

In the following decade, several other testosterones' derivatives were also synthesized, such as stanozolol (Winstrol), methenolone (Primobolan), mesterolone (Proviron), oxymetholone (Anadrol) and drostanolone (Masterone). All of them were serving medical purposes, fighting specific symptoms (anemia, hypogonadism, muscle wasting, osteopenia, breast cancer).

During the "Cold War" era (early 50's-late 80's) in the former Eastern Bloc (East Germany, Soviet Union, Bulgaria, China and N.Korea later) the science of doping was consolidated in order to promote communism.The "Cold War" era was a conflict between East and West in Olympic Games.

It was well known the alleged "breakfast of the champions", the pharmaceutical oral 17 alkylated AAS Turinabol (DDR).This AAS was quite familiar with the Russian Dianabol (methandienone-methandrostenolone) ortheBulgarianBionabol.

Although it was suspected that AAS were being used systematically by athletes, testing methods were insufficiently developed.In 1975, the International Olympic Committee (IOC) banned the use of steroids in Olympic competition and in 1976 steroid testing was conducted for the first time at the Montreal Olympics.

Some decades later, in the mid 90s, the extensive doping abuse of GDR was exposed in documents. Type of drugs, doses, programs and proper withdrawal timing prior to the games were revealed. Almost 70% of athletes, who joined the Munich 1972 Olympics, were chemically enhanced.

When health problems appeared, former champions pressed charges against their trainers and physicians for non-reversible medical side effects.

Bodybuilding

After the Berlin's wall fall and the end of the Cold War era, gurus and coaches abandoned Europe to immigrate into the USA, asking for political asylum. Their "knowhow" strategies, along with the advanced technology available from the Americans, developed new methods of doping and created the advanced gene doping with applications in the genetic material (DNA).Synthetic forms, recombinant Human Growth Hormone (r-HGH), insulin-like growth factor 1(r-IGF-1) and erythropoietin (r-EPO) were the new weapons of performance enhancement drugs (PED's).

At 2000 r-EPO was speculated to be widely abused by endurance athletes (distance running,cycling, race-walking, cross-country skiing, triathlons) and sprinters occasionally in Sydney Olympics.

Some elite cyclists in the Tour de France, including Lance Armstrong, admitted to using r-EPO.

At 2003 BALCO scandalwasrevealed inthe USA.Tetrahydrogestrinone (THG) a17-alkylated AAS per os, the first non detected drugknown as "The clear". It was manufactured as a performance enhancer not for medical purposes.Victor Conte was the manager of Bay Area Laboratory Cooperation (BALCO). Tetrahydrogestrinonewas an anabolic steroid in liquid form, with progestational activity and high liver toxicity. Its origin comes from gestrinone (a progesterone's derivative, a steroid prescribed against endometriosis i.e. inner wall uterus thickening), being added four (4) hydrogen (H2) atoms.Marion Jones & Tim Montgomery were convicted and sent in prisonas a result of perjury.

It was the first time where athletes were suspended, without being tested positive, through numerousemails that ensured their use.

There have been many outbreaks at the Olympic Games still standing, as well as haunted suspicious WR or OR that have been broken but later rescinded by the IOC (10.49 sec & 10.54 sec, 21.54 sec) by Florence Griffith Joiner (USA-RIP 1998).In 1988 at Seoul Olympics there was an extensive abuse of AAS (stanozolol-Ben Johnson's scandal, 100m final 9.79 sec).There were also suspicions that Florence Griffith Joyner (Flo-Jo) records were the result of using steroids or other PED's (HGH), since performance had improved dramatically over a short period of time. Besides, her retirement in 1989 followed Ben Johnson's scandal over doping. When Flo Jo died at the age of 38 years, her heart was enlarged, consistent with cardiomyopathy from HGH abuse.

At 1996 Atlanta games, creatine monohydrate was the miraculous new supplement.

The 2000 Sydney Olympics belonged to r-EPO, which was not yet able to get under control.Until the 2004 Olympic Games in Athens, r-HGH was the undetected weapon of athletes.

DOPING-ANTIDOPING STRATEGIES

Doping at the Olympic Games will always be a step ahead of the anti-doping control, despite the large amounts of money invested by the IOC, trying to fight it. Nevertheless I do firmly believe that performance improvement is a result of the evolution of technology, expertise and coaching. The viewers-spectators would not fill the stadiums, nor pay for expensive tickets, if they were to watch poor performances. Consequently, the sponsors would not offer big contracts-motives to the athletes. Therefore, everything comes under and is a product of commercialization.

The concept of doping is reduced to science, where talent combined with hard work, can break records. Surprisingly, when they asked a hundred American athletes if they would use doping to win an Olympic gold medal. At the same time, they informed them that five years later they would pass away, asa result of health complications and side effects of the drugs. Surprisingly, 55% responded positively, that they would use it. This indicates that, the motive of vanity and ephemeral glorious life is indeed big.

As someone once said, it is better to live 50 years as a tiger, than live 100 as a lamb. The issue starts from the audience, and whether they want to watch supremeperformances, smashing world records, or go back to the olive clone and the spirit of Baron Pierre de Coubertin "participation is more important than victory".

Years ago, Stavros Hatzos MD, who practices in sport medicine, wrote in his book about doping: "Doping gives you credit, while narcotics discredit you. The Olympic medalist meets the President, in the salons, while the drug addict is dying helpless in the streets. The champion is highly paid, while the drug user is starving to death. However, while doping, which is a must for the commercialized highly competitive championships, is reprehensible and despicable, narcotics arestill popular among parties of the high VIP society". Contradictory phenomena of a hypocritical society that weighs situations with different standards.

Once the bitter, but authoritative sports journalist Philip Syrigos (RIP) stated the following paradox thing: "it shouldn't be just the athletes who go up the podium anymore, but the doctors with the syringes and the pills they provided them with." It was a radical statement, partly true.

But as in any sport – mainly individual – we should not overlook the factors of talent and hard work-dedication. And finally, as the Olympic spirit ended up being, the athletes are pushed to always strive for more (faster, higher, stronger), who in fact are the victims of a corrupt commercializedsystem. Starting from the society and the particular government. The propaganda of the former communist regimes for direct promotion of the country, through the Olympic Games was well known (Cuba, China, Soviet Union-CCCP, East Germany-DDR, Bulgaria, and Korea).

According to Chris Tzekostrack and field coach, "doped is the one gets busted as positive, at the W.A.D.A./U.S.A.D.A scheduled control process". However, according to physician Stavros Hatzos MD,"being aware of the half life of a particular substance, plus the scheduled date of the urine drug test, we can withdraw from using it". This practically refutes the claim of the former athletics coach, while it essentially confirms that only unannounced doping tests are effective. When referring to the half life of a substance, we practically mean the necessary time that is required for the metabolism and elimination, half of the administrated dose.

Some factors that contribute to the metabolism of a substance are: 1) hydration state, 2) metabolic rate, 3) workout intensity, 4) subcutaneous body fat percentage.

According to the recent methods, the metabolites of AAS are now detected. Therefore, a substance may be inactive in the body for a certain period of time, which practically translates to minimal benefits for the athlete. However, months later its metabolites will betray for its use.

During the anti doping testing process, other than the metabolites of a substance, it is also carried out a hormonal measurement of the testosterone/epitestosterone ratio, which should be below six(6). Therefore, if someone uses testosterone within small amounts, T/E ratio will predict any exogenous administration.

AAS in tablet form (per os)

Oxymetholone: 8 hrs

Oxandrolone: 9 hrs

Methandrostenolone: 6 hrs

Stanozolol: 9 hrs

Injectable AAS

Nandrolone decaonate: 14 days

Equipoise: 14 days

Trenbolone acetate: 3 days

Methenolone enanthate: 10 days

Testosterone cypionate: 12 days

Testosterone enanthate: 10 days

Testosterone propionate: 4 days

Testosterone suspension: 24 hrs

Stanozolol: 24 hrs

The biological passport is an advanced detection method, with which the athlete literally getsfiled. Urinesamples are kept for almost a decade. So in case he/she used a banned but not detected substance back then, that s detectable now, he/she looses medals and trophies.

Apart from the classical methods of substance and metabolites detection, an athlete who uses doping will give themselves away by certain laboratory (biochemical, hormonal) hematological tests. An experienced biopathologist and sports medicine doctor, can recognize whether the athlete has used doping.

The values that will be corrupted are the following:

Hematocrit:

It is known that the AAS promote the process of erythrocytosis and cause the rise in hemoglobin. The reason why this happens is that EPO is produced by the kidney which stimulates the red bone marrow.

Tsansaminases:

AAS (mainly 17 alkaloids) are hepatotoxic and increase the liver function tests (ALT-SGPT/AST-SGOT), a reaction of the liver parenchyma to their metabolism. This is first stage, known as pharmaceutical hepatitis.

Lipoproteins-Lipids:

The biosynthesis of lipoproteins of high and low density (HDL/LDL) is made up in the liver parenchyma. When the liver suffers from AAS use, their values get altered, resulting in the disturbance of the atheromatic index and fraction (HDL drops/LDL elevates).

Coagulation time:

The INP, APTT are clotting factors, synthesized by liver. When the liver is under strength, both the INP and the APTT increase their values, while hemostatic mechanisms get disturbed, resulting in the prolonged of coagulation (bleeding time).

Luteinising (LH) &follicle stimulating hormone(FSH):

The process of homeostasis keeps a balance and whenever there is an exogenous use of AAS, the hypothalamus and the pituitary close the operation "switch" and the HPTA gets suppressed.

Total, free testosterone:

It is reasonable that their absolute values in serum will be increased, because of the exogenous administration of AAS, which are synthetic derivatives of testosterone.

Somatomedin C:

During an exogenous use of somatomedin, the liver produces the insulin-like growth factor, also known as IGF1.This is a reliable method of using a growth hormone, reaching its peak metabolism, within two hours.

HOW ATHLETES GET DOPED

A large percentage of athletes are forced to use PEDS because of their high competitive and paid professional championship. In fact, athletes play hide and seek in their goal to become more competitive. This, in part seems realistic, as requirements are large.

The doping methods used are the following:

1) Use of unknown substance

This method essentially constitutes the ideal doping, as there are no reagents for detecting it. These are substances that are not indicated for therapeutic administration of specific diseases, but are custom made in the laboratory for use as ergogenic substances.

Of course, with the existence of the biological passport, substances that are undetectable for a specific period of time can later be detected when the reagents are known and manufactured.

Thus, when an athlete made a record using a particular substance unknown to him on the day of the game, he would now be positive and be removed from the medal. This is because the passport holds a urine sample of a distinguished athlete and the biological samples are analyzed over time.

An example was tetrahedrogestrinone (THG), manufactured by Patrick Arnold and BALCO. Before 2003 it was not detected, but ten years later records and medals were removed by athletes who had used it at that time.

2) Use of testosterone- epitestosterone

Testosterone is a natural substance for the body, unlike its synthetic derivatives (AAS).

Therefore an athlete who is using testosterone is more difficult to detect than the metabolites of synthetic steroids, which the body does not produce. An athlete can claim either a hormonal condition, or specific conditions that increase his testosterone to higher normal levels.

Exogenous use of testosterone (T) is predicted by the concentration of epitestosterone (E), a substance that maintains a close correlation of concentration with the basic androgen. This is the T / E ratio, which should not exceed six (6). These two hormones are closely related and correlated with the body.

In the case of exogenous use of testosterone (e.g., injectable form), the concentration of epitestosterone is not increased at the same time, and thus their ratio exceeds the defined limit. In order for athletes to conceal the exogenous use of testosterone, they should keep the hormone ratio within the permitted limit. One way is the appropriate dose that will not disturb their proportion. Another method is the parallel administration of both hormones in the correct ratio. This method was the case of the famous "cream" by BALCO at the time of the scandal in 2003.

3) Use of beta-human chorionic gonadotropin

This peptide is produced by the placenta during the first weeks of pregnancy. It has the potential to increase luteinizing hormone (mimic) and then endogenous testosterone production. It was observed that female athletes who had increased testosterone in their first month of pregnancy did better. In men, this hormone helps the endogenous production of testosterone, but also epitestosterone.

But beta- hCG is readily detected in the urine - this method is used as a diagnostic component of pregnancy. Still this substance is on the list of prohibited substances of the World Anti-Doping Federation (WADA/USADA).

4) Using a mask

Masks are agents used to "conceal" or "cover up" other doping agents. They are not ergogenic compounds, but interfere with the metabolic rate and excretion of substances by the body. Tests are usually done on the metabolites of the substance rather than the substance itself. Masks have the property of changing the metabolism of a substance used and of modifying its metabolites. Other masks have the property of blocking the excretion of a substance from the kidneys. While others have the potential to dilute the concentration of the substance to undetectable levels.

- Probenecid is one of the masks.

It is primarily used in treating gout and hyperuricemia. Probenecid inhibits the tubular resorption of uric acid, thereby increasing uric acid excretion in the urine and decreasing serum uric acid levels. It has the property of inhibiting the renal excretion of the glucuronide steroid molecule, one of the major metabolites of steroid molecules in the urine. But the substance probenecid as a mask is a forbidden substance in the WADA / USADA list.

- 5α reductase inhibitors are antiandrogens that inhibit the reduction of testosterone to dihydrotestosterone (DHT). Finasteride and dutasteride decrease the androgen DHT concentration. They are therefore used when the assay procedures focus on the detection of DHT and the remaining steroid derivatives.

- Diuretics

These substances are administered for the dilution of urine, leading to lower-undetectable levels of the forbidden substance. Of course, even sparse urine concentration, either with diuretics or with high water consumption, alters the specific weight of the urine, which is not permitted. Therefore, these tests require a morning urine sample where the concentration of all substances is the result of the overnight renal metabolic process and the specific weight of the urine is increased.

- Ketoconazole

Ketoconazole is a synthetic imidazole antifungal drug used primarily to treat fungal infections by inhibiting ergosterol biosynthesis. In humans, at high dosages (>800 mg/day), it inhibits the activity of several enzymes necessary for the conversion of cholesterol to steroid hormones such as testosterone, thus interferes with the metabolism of doping substances. It has the potential to alter the testosterone-epitestosterone (T / E) ratio and therefore make it difficult to detect exogenous testosterone.

5) Use of a substance on medical advice

It is known that PEDS are used in medicine for therapeutic purposes in certain diseases. Hypogonadism, anemia, muscular cachexia, osteoporosis, endometriosis, angioedema, multiple sclerosis, asthma, allergic rhinitis are some of the conditions.

AAS are mainly used to treat hormonal disorders, while stimulants (sympathomimetics, adrenergic) in respiratory diseases. If the athlete is examined by a physician and needs a certain substance, then the use of this agent is allowed only within acceptable limits. The coach should be informed by his athlete, who should also inform the respective federation.

Sometimes athletes choose this kind of "legally doping" method,however they fail to justify it on time.There was a case of a Greek female golden Olympic champion at the 2004 games. Initially she was busted for being positive, by using a beta- 2 agonist. Later she claimed, that salboutamol found in her system, was part of her asthmatic treatment.

PEDS IN MODERN SOCIETY

The androgen anabolic steroids (AAS) along with growth hormone (somatropin) can become the elixir of youth, when we use them sensibly, wisely, in moderation and sparingly. The joints hurt less, the muscles get toned resulting in the decrease of the belly fat, the skin becomes more flexible, self-confidence increases and libido improves. Bones get stronger, injures heal faster.Rejuvenation is achieved by growth hormone somatropin.

However, as there is always a flip side to every coin, irrational use and years of abuse can be fatal, sort of a time bomb. Hepatocellular carcinoma, acute renal failure, prostate tumor, psychotic behaviors, bipolar disorder, acne, infertility, sleep apnea, heart enlargement, hypertension, diabetes, carpal tunnel syndrome are some of the complications.

AAS were not manufactured by physicians for athletes.Their purpose was to treat certain diseases and syndromes under specific dosages.However, coaches and athletes took advantage of their collateral effects related to athletic performance and abused them extensively (10x times more).

If an athlete is into bodybuilding and wishes for longevity, he also needs to remain healthy. And this does not reflect only on the musculoskeletal lesions and injuries, but also in the well functioning of the internal organs and their metabolism. This directly implies the lifestyle, the avoidance of harmful habits and using common sense. For example, one cannot use drugs that stress heart's function while on a steroid cycle, nor consume alcoholic beverages lashing even more the already stressed liver. But also someone who is hospitalized or under medical supervision, has to listen carefully to his doctor's advice. Common sense dictates the sense of self-preservation, which in simple words means that one should not commit suicide.

One of the reasons why chronic steroids users remain addicted is the fact that, apart from the dramatic improvement of their appearance (muscularity increase, subcutaneous fat reduction, muscle strength, physical strength), steroids affect mental sphere and emotional status.

Soon after stopping their use, there are immediate symptoms such as depression, musculoskeletal pain, decline of physical performance, sarcopenia, libido reduction, belly fat increase. Therefore, steroids users soon resort to new cycles that actually perpetuate the existing problem and create a vicious cycle in the whole issue.

New drug combinations, larger doses, longer treatments are the alternative "solutions". The addiction to psychoactive substances like caffeine, amphetamine, ephedrine HCL act on the mental sphere and linked to euphoria (well being state), along with performance enhancing properties (analgesia, thermogenesis, mental focus, cognition).Therefore, it is obvious that all these substances become very addictive.

AAS are literally the narcotics of sports, in case their use becomes uncontrolled, without medical monitoring.AAS, growth factors and stimulants are potentially considered as a public health issue.

Personally, I do strongly believe that this issue is likely multifactorial.

Bodybuilding

Firstly, it is undeniable that these drugs are highly effective and definitely work; they improve dramatically performance and body image.

Secondly, the social standards in our modern era dictate the masculine sculpted physique.

An "alpha male" consists of broad shoulders, strong arms, massive thighs, a herculean chest, with a tight midsection. This was even illustrated in action films. We can observe the dramatic shift of action heroes from the 50s era to the 80s. In other words, the transition from Steve Reeves and Kirk Douglas to Arnold Schwarzenegger and Sylvester Stallone.

There was an interesting study, conducted at Harvard University, by Harrison Pope MD. Individuals who had made heavy and extensive abuse of AAS/PEDs, had the tendency to avoid pleasant social activities, like swimming, sports where they could take their shirts off, simply because they had very high standards for themselves. In other words, they had to be perfectly fit, in order to reveal their physique. The same athletes had also the syndrome of bulking-mania, or muscle dysmorphia. This whole narcissistic mentality, is also named as "Adonis complex".

That is an excessive dedication that resembles of an obsession with their body image and the way others look at them. The concept of physical deformity refers to the fact that a bodybuilder, although he is huge, he is never satisfied because of his insecurity. Essentially, this is the diametrically opposite mental disorder of anorexia nervosa.

We live in a society with a highly demanding lifestyle where chemical enhancement occurs on a daily basis. Recreational use of stimulants (cocaine, amphetamines), in order to perform at the gym and improve cognitive function at work. Barbiturates (diazepam), taken at night to relief stress and enhance sleeping process.Both of which classes of drugs are highly addictive and potentially fatal. CNS stimulants such as caffeine,ephedrine and clenbuterol hightly abused from bodybuilders and track athletes,are capable of heart attack and stroke. On the other hand,barbiturates can suppress respiratory center and lead to sleep apnea and even death. Moreover, 5PDEi are used even by young men who want to perform better in bed and minimize any erectile dysfunction. Furthermore,F1 and moto GP drives but also F16 pilots may use modafinil in order to boost cognitive ability and state of alert,improving nootropic response. While cops and university student use amphetamines during late shifts to sustain overnight work. Snipers also use beta 2 blockers for stability during shooting practice. Even artists like actors or singers sniff cocaine in order to perform better on stage.Similarly a hard worker may smoke weed to chill out and take a nap.

In the bottom oine everyone is cheating on a daily basis in every aspect of his life. Why the heck someone who wills to improve his physical appearance and boost his self esteem,or even his strength and the gym,is still considered as a cheater or a villain? Its about time finally to face the facts without any prejudice and suspicion.

THE SIGNIFICANCE OF MEDICAL PREVENTION IN BODYBUILDING

Bodybuilding is impressive, but is also a double-edged sword, when it is not consisted with the requirements of knowledge-knowhow and prevention. You should not blame the drugs in case you use them carelessly, or if you stack carelessly different compounds.

The contradictory and paradoxical with the use of chemical enhancementis that while you improve your external appearance, at the same moment, you risk your health. Conversely, when you cease using drugs, your physique starts to flaw, but your health starts getting better and laboratory tests improve.

Each doctor is obliged to tell to his patients how to preserve well being. The fact that bodybuilders decide not to follow it, is due to their vanity, weaknesses and personal choices.

The sport of bodybuilding involves a risk, a craze, a vanity, all of which pose dangers in the long term, so exaggeration and the thought "the more is better" is not panacea and does not necessarily guarantee success. Side effects of a particular substance are dependent on various parameters, such as age, time of abuse, dosage, combination of performance enhancing drugs (PED's), life style, proper nutrition and supplementation, medical prevention rules and family history.

Time of abuse and dosage play a major role. This practically translates into either big doses for a small amount of period (shocking therapy), or small doses for prolonged duration. So, small doses of testosterone as TRT (hormone replacement) will offer a better libido, muscularity, skin elasticity, improved Bone

Mineral Density, improved self esteem and sexual drive, diminish of omental fat – midsection's fat reduction, resulting ultimately in a confidence boost as a way of life. But over time, there might be changes in the atherosclerotic profile – fraction (HDL/LDL), inflammation of the prostate gland (BPH) because of the reduction to DHT, androgenic alopecia (MPB), hair growth on the back – shoulders, thickening of heart's left ventricle. That's the reason why regular medical monitoring by measuring the values of PSA/FREE PSA, biochemical serum tests and echocardiography are required. The same applies to the anti-aging somatropin(HGH) as well. Even small doses of 4 IU daily in five years time, it is possible to cause excrescences in the abdominal region due to visceral enlargement (small and large intestine, liver, spleen) irrespective of the use of insulin. The only difference is that while some things are potentially reversible, others are not, such as the cardiomegaly, acromegalyand the possibility of tumor genesis (colon cancer).

You don't have to make brief abuses to get ill. Even minimal doses for prolonged periods may result in similar medical issues. Overall lifestyle and the prevention rules play a major role. Lifestyle includes a healthy diet, low in sugar-refined carbohydrates saturated-trans fats and salt, with a variety of fruits and vegetables, fiber-rich whole grains and low-fat dairy products.For overall cardiovascular health a regular (5 times per week) cardiovascular physical activity is recommended. Also cessation of smoking, moderate use of alcohol and avoidance of narcotics are mandatory preventive approaches. Before the onset, during and after the end of an AAS/PEDs cycle, the user has the obligation to undergo specific blood teststo evaluate his general medical condition. This is crucial firstly to determine the user's current health and risks before any cycle is initiated, then to assess the direct impact of the AAS/PEDs use and finally to evaluate the distortion or restoration of original state of good health.We all have a specified genetic predisposition (DNA), which largely determines our genetic limits and our standards. Anabolic androgenic steroids (AAS) do not kill instantly, or at least not in a few hours. On the contrary, 30mg of benzodiazepam can lead to a coma, due to respiratory center suppression. Also 5gr of salicylic acid (aspirin) will lead to lead to gastric mucosa bleeding and ulcer. Impressively, a high dosage of potassium can be lethal, as a result of ventricular fibrillation.

The most dangerous drugs in bodybuilding are:

1) insulin,

2) diuretics and

3) CNS stimulants.

These medications can lead respectively to lethal:

1) hypoglycemic coma,

2) hypovolemic shock and severe heart arrhythmia,

3) aneurysm rupture, leading to hemorrhagic stroke and acute myocardial infarction, in other words heart attack.

Chemical enhancement with PEDs receives a negative propaganda. It's impressive that the majority of those who use PED's are not professional athletes, but mainly recreational or amateur athletes.

AAS/PEDs are not the first choice drugs on pharmacy shelves. They are specialized drugs, manufactured and prescribed for the treatment of certain diseases (hypogonadism, anemia, osteoporosis, muscle weakness, angioedema, AIDS cachexia, breast cancer) and used under medical prescription.

The legal status of AAS varies from country to country; some have stricter controls on their use or prescription than others, though in many countries they are not illegal. In U.S.A., AAS are currently listed as Class C controlled substances, same as barbiturates and opioids. As a former athlete, who competed at the bodybuilding nationals, I realized that the persecution against chemical enhancement resulted to withdraw specific steroids worldwide by legit pharmaceutical companies. Unfortunately, they were replaced by underground and illegal products (counterfeits). Contamination is easier to happen, since these chemicals do not obey to ISO standards for human use. Heavy metals and poor quality solvents (oils) are most likely to be presented. Of course under dosed solutions is also a highly possible case scenario.

CNS STIMULANTS

CLENBUTEROL HYDROCHLORIDE (Clenbuterol HCL)

It belongs to the class of b2 stimulants and it is sympathomimetic with adrenergic action.

It is used for asthma due to its ability to induce bronchodilation. This results in increased oxygen consumption (VO2max) by the tissues, which increases the combustions and the performance.

It also causes positive inotropic effect on the cardiac muscle-myocardium, with tachycardia, increased blood pressure, rapid breathing-respiration, sweating, hand tremors, insomnia, and restlessness.

Its complications – side effects include ischemic attacks with the appearance of angina pectoris (ischemic effect) because of vasoconstriction. Also arrhythmia, with the appearance of atrial fibrillation and ventricular tachycardia. Fibrillation is a form of cardiac arrhythmia, which in extreme cases can transform into ventricular fibrillation and cardiac arrest. Furthermore, intense sweating causes dehydration and hypokalemia (drop in potassium levels), causing muscle spasms – cramps. It also has a cardiotoxic effect on the myocardium, with necrotic effects-scar tissue. Its ability to oxidize and catabolise fat is impressive, especially when combined with thyroxine (T4), or triiodothyronine (T3).

It's chronic abuse - due to the increase of the diastolic pressure - may lead to left ventricular hypertrophy (LVH) of myocardium.

The disadvantage of clenbuterol's use is the fast saturation of the receptors.

This is why, its administration should not be continuous, but ceased every two days (48hrs) and afterwards the dose should be increased by half, until one can get the desired results. The maximum safety dosage should not exceed 80mg daily.

Its half-life reaches approximately around 36 hours, while it can be detected even up to five days after one has quit from using it. Another way to unblock the saturation of the receptors is the use of a substance named ketotifen (medically prescribed and administrated for allergic rhinitis – asthma).

Clenbuterol HCL is available either in tablet, or in liquid (syrup) form. Recently, it was released in injectable form, so it can be administratedsubcutaneously. It is advised to avoid taking it after noon, because it causes insomnia.

Clenbuterol is occasionally used during post cycle therapy (PCT to keep our metabolic rate high, when the androgens clear the system and fat oxidation drops dramatically. Also, clenbuterol hydrochloride has a positive effect on the increase of thyroxin's levels and thyroid gland metabolism. Finally, by inhibiting the adrenocorticotropic hormone (ACTH), it helps reducing the catabolic cortisol during a PCT.

An alternative to clenbuterol is the substance salbutamol (b2 – stimulant), that comes in spray form and is ideal just before a sports activity, or even before getting on stage. It is more effective for asthmatic crises, since it acts locally on bronchi receptors. It has a faster half life though.

Clenbuterol is banned from WADA,unlike salbutamol.The reason is the fact its more effective in fat burning and more potent in elevating blood pressure.However its less effective in terms of bronchodilation under asthmatic crisis.On the other hand,salbutamol is less effective in beta oxidation,but far superior as anti asthmatic medication.

EPHEDRINE HYDROCHLORIDE (EPHEDRINE HCL)

It is administrated for allergic rhinitis (runny nose) and it belongs to the sympathomimetic central nervous system (CNS) stimulants, with adrenergic action. It stimulates b2 receptors, but with a smaller affinity on the receptors of the upper respiratory tract (trachea, bronchi). It has the ability to cause vasoconstriction, leading to blood pressure increase, through the production of adrenaline – epinephrine. It has similar effects with clenbuterol HCL.

It is combined as a stack, along with caffeine and aspirin – salicylic acid. Therefore, they act synergistically as catalysts (ECA: 25mg ephedrine, 250mg caffeine, 300mg aspirin), thus increasing the body temperature.

However, in extreme cases this may lead to hyperpyrexia (an increase of body core temperature), or lower grade fever and reduction of the feeling of fatigue and physical pain. That resembles the action of amphetamines. The use of ECA stack increases dramatically systemic blood pressure, which is a serious contraindication for hypertensive patients.

Ephedrine alkaloids bring a state of euphoria to the CNS. This may develop into hypomania and restlessness feeling. Insomnia is very likely to occur, due to CNS overstimulation. The pupils of the eyes are contracted and peripheral vasoconstriction in limbs is responsible for poor vascularity.

As a result, it's a not a wise idea to use ephedrine HCL prior to sexual intercourse. Ephedrine causes peripheral vasoconstriction in the cavernous bodies of the penis. Occasionally, it gives an acute pain to perineum, which implies the stimulation of prostate gland.

Using ephedrine in a bodybuilding show will hinder vascularity and diminish the pumping effect of veins. It is advised to be used before cardiovascular training, on an empty stomach, in order to maximize both intensity and fat burning process (beta oxidation of fatty acids).

Ephedrine's action starts within half an hour, the peak of its action is within an hour of use, and its half life is approximately estimated around three hours.

Ephedrine HCL is a very useful tool when dieting, since it suppresses appetite and gives that satiety feeling.

YOHIMBINE HYDROCHLORIDE

The yohimbe bark herb stimulates the a2 adrenergic receptors. It causes positive inotropic, chronotropic action, through sympatheticomimetic effect.

Twenty years ago, its use was an alternative supplementation for erectile dysfunction, due to vascular issues. Yohimbine HCL - unlike clenbuterol and ephedrine HCL - causes peripheral vasodilation and vascular permeability. This solves the erectile dysfunctional problems in corpus cavernosum (cavernous bodies) of the penis. At the same time, it prevents the return of blood to the heart through the venous system. Yohimbine was widely used, way before **nitric oxide** (NO) production drugs were manufactured.

In the sport of bodybuilding, Yohimbine HCL (yohimbe bark) is an ideal tool for boosting vascularity before getting on stage. Moreover, it enhances the process of beta oxidation and lipolysis in subcutaneous tissue. Its action is thermogenetic and therefore increases the **Basal Metabolic Rate(**BMR), leading to fat catabolism.

CAFFEINE

Caffeine belongs to the class of methylxanthines. It increases the aerobic capacity in a manner similar to the one of clenbuterol hydrochloride (bronchodilator- leading to the increase of VO2max). It does not belong to the same class of substances (b-2 stimulants), but has the ability to cause bronchodilation, so in doses >3mg/kg acts an alternative solution for the treatment of paroxysmal asthmatic crisis.

Caffeine also stimulates smooth muscle layer of small intestine, which is regulated by the autonomic nervous system, so soon after we drink coffee with breakfast, an urge for defecation starts.

A fatal overdose of caffeine for a bodybuilder with a body weight of 100kg, is approximately around 10gr in a single dose (100mg/kg); while lethal levels in blood are found at around 80mg. Death occurs from cardiac arrest due to ventricular tachycardia – fibrillation.

The intoxication of caffeine causes irritability-restlessness, tremor-trembling, rapid breathing-respiration, sweating, headaches, diarrhea syndromes, precordial chest pain and delirium.

The abuse and addiction to caffeine is the most widespread and legal way of chemical enhancement, worldwide, on a daily basis.

Caffeine is able to pass through blood brain barrier and placenta.

Caffeine acts synergistically as a catalyst to ephedrine hydrochloride and enhances beta oxidation of fatty acids, consequently lipolysis of the subcutaneous tissue. The peak of its concentration occurs within an hour, while its half-life is estimated around four hours. Proper dosage is estimated at 3mg/kg of body weight (300mg for a 100kg athlete). Even larger dosages (5mg/kg), increase the maximum strength and training intensity. At normal doses, caffeine has effects on learning and memory, improving reaction time, alertness, attention and concentration.

Caffeine is quite often combined with painkillers, such as paracetamol and multiplies the masking pain effect. It is also an antidote for a hangover crisis and migraine episode.

THYROXINE T4 (THYROXINE)

It is a hormone produced in the thyroid gland, which determines the basal metabolic rate and is directly related to the weight loss-gain. It has a lipolytic ability, but also muscle catabolism as an adverse effect. Its administration should be done with extra caution, since the HPT axis gets easily disturbed and after a certain point the situation is irreversible. Tapering is a good way to get off from thyroid supplementation. Its abuse results in irregular heartbeat-tachycardia, insomnia, sweating, exophthalmos (eyes bulging), restlessness, muscle catabolism and regain of weight, as soon as someone stop its use. It's a typical rebound effect, since BMR drops.

For proper gland's health, it is advised to consume iodized salt, or even iodine in the form of kelp, along with the amino acid L-tyrosine, which is involved in biosynthesis of T3 (triiodothyronine). T3 is more potent than T4 (thyroxine), having a shorter half-life. Therefore, it should be used twice daily, unlike thyroxine. Considering that T4 makes T3, when we use thyroid hormones, if we do not grant T4 – but only T3, progressively its stocks will get decreased. Therefore, it is better to use T4, with which T3 will be formed as well. Of course, its combination is even stronger, but poses risks for the myocardium and muscle catabolism with prolonged overdose and without progressive reduction (for proper balance of the thyroid hormone TSH). The axis of the thyroid hormone is very sensitive and the TSH should be set in the middle of the normal range values. Hypo/hyperthyroidism is an outcome of various different evaluations (TSH, T4, FT4, T3, FT3, ANTI-TPO, ANTI-TG). Athletes have ended up being hypothyroid, due to the extensive abuse of T3.

AMPHETAMINES

Amphetamines belong to the psychotropic sympathomimetic stimulants. They stimulate the adrenergic receptors in myocardium and central nervous system (CNS). Their properties are similar to the ones of the alkaloid ephedrine, including euphoria-hypomania, anorexia-satiety, thermogenesis, increased fatty acid oxidation – lipolysis, alertness-restlessness, sleeplessness-insomnia, tachycardia-increased heart rate, arrhythmias -palpitations, tremors-trembling and tachypnea- increased respiration. They are highly effective for beta oxidation because they induce brown adipose tissue (located beneath the scapula), the most important organ for non-shivering thermogenesis.

In medicine, they were initially prescribed and administrated for the clinical phenomenon of narcolepsy, where the individual shows drowsiness and psychosomatic fatigue with changes in their sleep schedule. In modern medicine, amphetamines were medically used as a method to suppress hunger and appetite, or even to boost BMR and fat burning effect.

Amphetamines are highly addictive, as several people have made extensive uses of it, like soldiers in the World War II, Afghanistan, Gulf War, or even police officers in the US during late shifts. Amphetamines were widely spread among university students in Europe and USA.

The reason why amphetamines are highly addictive is due to the increase of neurotransmitter dopamine. Dopamine is associated with the feeling of reward, initiative and self-confidence. Moreover, they increase the concentration of neurotransmitter serotonin linked with the feeling of joy and happiness. They also affect the limbic system dealing with emotional status.

In sports, amphetamines are widely used by track athletes in explosive sports (speed, throws, jumps), but also athletes who demand stamina and endurance (tennis, soccer, volleyball, cycling).

They provide alert and increase of fatigue threshold. Motor drivers (F1 and Moto GP) for improved concentration, alertness and focus.

The side effects of its use are nausea, vomiting, diarrhea syndromes, palpitations – arrhythmias, hypomania and emotional instability.The peak of amphetamines action occurs within an hour.

ANABOLIC HORMONES

SOMATROPIN – GROWTH HORMONE (HGH)

Growth Hormone (HGH) is a polypeptide composed of hundreds of amino acids (191). It is produced in infancy and adolescence by the anterior pituitary gland (adenohypophysis).

The synthetic form of HGH is produced in the laboratory by the method of recombinant DNA from E.Coli. Until 1985, GH treatment using human pituitary growth hormones extracted from deceased individuals or chimpanzees had a significant risk of transmission bovine spongiform encephalopathy(Creutzfeld Jakob disease).

The agents that promote HGH secretion are:

1)   fasting (low insulin – high glucagon),

2)   L-arginine,L-ornithine, lysine, clonidine (against hypertension), L-Dopa (against Parkinson's disease),

3)   multi-joint free-weight exercises such as dead lifts, squats and night sleep 11pm-7am,

4)   lactate production during anaerobic activity,

5)   estrogenic environment.

HGH is also released during the REM (rapid eye movement) phase of night sleep (11pm-7am).

Somatropin acts synergistically with testosterone, insulin, thyroxin and high caloric diets. The cells that constitute the 191 amino acids are activated by GHRH peptide in the hypothalamus.HGH in puberty has the ability to promote all cells and promote tissue growth, through hyperplasia. However in adults, hypertrophic phenomena occur instead.

Somatropin's hypertrophic effect is stimulated by somatomedin C (insulin growth factor or IGF-1), a hormone homologous to proinsulin. All organs seem to respond to it, except those that are in closed cavities and their expansion is impossible (eyeballs, brain). All visceral organs though, including soft tissues (lips, ears, tongue, gums) are overfed because of the remodeling – proliferation of cells (mitotic cellular divisions).Epidermis (skin) also gets thicker, while tendons, joints, articular capsules, cartilage are regenerated by the connective tissue collagen synthesis (chondroblastic activity).Effect on myocardial growth is evident, leading after chronic abuse to cardiomegaly, cardiomyopathy (HGH-induced), increased rate of cardiovascular disease and progressive heart failure.

Muscle hypertrophy caused by the use of HGH, implies the hyperplasia of all tissues.The elbows and the chin protrude, the forehead grows, the jaw widens (dentures – braces), hands and feet grow as well. It is the characteristic acromegaly after the end of puberty. This is however something that former chemist of BALCO & Ketosports,Patrick Arnold refuses.He supports that after the closure of epipheseal plates,hyperplastic phenomena don't occur at least in skeletal-contractile-sriated muscle tissue.Unlike the author of Anabolics book,William Llewellyn and Muscular Development writer Dave Palumbo who in fact both support the opposite.

r- HGH's huge benefits involve anti-aging at low doses (2 IU daily) and the mobilization of fat, at double dose (4 IU), while at doses of 8-16 IU, is an excellent muscle growth agent. It contributes to positive nitrogen balance, by the entry of amino acids into muscle cell, while it has an adverse effect on insulin. Therefore, it releases glucose in the circulation (gluconeogenesis in liver) and free fatty acids, contributing to the lipolysis of the subcutaneous tissue, which antagonizes the effect of insulin.

The indicated doses per kg of body weight concern only young children with hypopituitarism- dwarfism. In every product, quantities are measured in mg. The ratio between mg and international units (IU) is 1/3. Therefore, 12mg of pharmaceutical recombinant somatropin is substantially 36 IU.The leading pharmaceutical growth hormones are Saizen, Genotropin, Norditropin, Serostim, and Humatrope.

HGH has a half life of 30 minutes, while the peak of its action is reached at 120 minutes. Within 36 hours, the metabolic activity is ceased. When it is administered before sleep, we sabotage its natural secretion during the REM stage. It is better to be administrated twice a day, in the morning on a fasted state and post training. The ideal time to use r-HGH, is when the stomach is empty and hunger is present (low insulin – high glucagon). After the use of r-HGH, one should not consume carbohydrates for at least half an hour, as long as the half life of HGH exists. Otherwise, the insulin release from pancreas will hinder its metabolic activity. In other words, using r-HGH requires hunger and not carbohydrates. This is possible early AM, first thing in the morning, when the serum glucose levels are low. Its subcutaneous use extends the absorption by one hour compared to the intramuscular which gets instantly absorbed, as it enters directly into the blood stream. However, we diminish the local fat oxidation effect.

Measuring IGF-1 & IGF1-BP3 are methods in order to verify r-HGH authenticity. With the exogenous use of the HGH, liver releases IGF1.

The measuring of IGF-1 should be made in half an hour (half-life). Normally, we should observe hyperglycemia, as HGH releases glucose in circulation from liver (gluconeogenesis).Aching of bones and joints is evidence that the effect is active.

HGH tends to reduce the natural production of thyroxin. This occurs because it favors convertion of thyroxine to triodothyronine (T4=>T3). As a result of it, it is advised to be combined with the smallest dose of T4 (25mg thyroxin), as long as the treatment lasts.

Chronic abuse of somatropin causes hypothyroidism (increase of the TSH -thyroid stimulating hormone).Hypothyroidism also appears in the form of nodular goiter in patients with pituitary adenoma, acromegaly and gigantism.In other words, a patient with anterior pituitary adenoma has similar symptoms to a chronic r-HGH abuser. Apparently, administration of T4 is necessary in both cases. In pituitary adenoma and gigantism, nodular goiter, abnormal glucose tolerance and diabetes mellitus type II (DM2) may coexist.

GH increases insulin resistance and consequently insulin action is reduced in both hepatic and extra hepatic tissues. So, the incidence of DM2 can be explained by the direct hyperglycaemic effects of excess HGH. As a counterweight, a small dose of insulin could be administrated, or metformin (<4 IU).

Other common symptoms that are observed along with r-HGH abuse and pituitary adenoma are acromegaly and arthritis. The latter is due to the friction of long bones epiphysis, as they grow.

Tibia and femur are the sites of epiphyseal plates from where a teenager grows. Bones that are also affected are humerus (brachium), radius and ulna (forearm) and the bones of wrist and ankle.

The braces that some athletes wear on their teeth, suggested the deformation of maxilla (upper jaw) and the thinning of front teeth, due to r-HGH use.

We often hear about athletes getting injured by the infamous "fatigue fractures". These take place, as a result of chronic abuse of somatropin. The explanation is that, as the muscles grow along the bones (tibia or fibula), they pull them. Consequently, periosteum of bones cracks, since it can't stand the forced pressure. This is something that occurs in combination with AAS abuse and repeated cushions (long jump, triple jump and high jump).

Carpal tunnel syndrome is another side effect. The wrist tendons get thicker due to fluid retention, which causes compression phenomena in the median nerve. Numbing of thumb and hand is a typical clinical syndrome. It can be treated surgically, by the incision and decompression of the carpal ligament.

Chronic abuse of somatropin has been implicated in neoplastic lesions, leukemia in particular. This happens because with doses >8 IU/24h, there is a release of IGF-1 from the liver.

The fundamental basis of tumor growth and carcinogenesis is the excessive proliferation of cells. HGH may stimulate tumor genes that undergo mutations and in combination with other factors, could lead to tumor genesis. Those, who have a family history of cancer, should firstly check their tumor markers (CEA, CA, 19-9, AFP). That is the reason why large doses of somatropin lead to tissue and muscle development, though the growth factor of insulin. In contrast, smaller doses <4 IU/24h, deal with lipolysis in particular.

Over time, somatropin users develop thickening of the upper airways (pharynx, larynx and glottis), resulting in partial obstruction and creation of sleep apnea. This is accompanied by snoring and awakening during sleep. This is reinforced by the cervical muscles overdeveloped. Subjects often complain for waking up with headache, poor concentration and memory, dysthymia-moodiness, derived from hypercapnia (CO_2 elevation). This is the result of hypoventilation and low oxygenation in brain.

Super heavy weight bodybuilders and strongmen have developed a neck circumference (> 45cm). The majority of them show the effect of obstructive sleep apnea, during which they snore in their sleep and wake up violently-abruptly. This phenomenon is due to the fact that the pharynx-upper respiratory tract has undergone hypertrophy from:

1) development of soft tissues, by r-HGH abuse

2) the strong muscular development of the cervical (trapezoid) and side cervical muscles (sternocleidomastoids).

Moreover, epiglottis relaxes during bedtime, due to the action of parasympathetic nervous system, thus resulting in that phenomenon.

HGH GUT

It is quite common the image of bodybuilding champions with a great protrusion of the abdomen.

There are several mechanisms that cause this phenomenon:

1) It is known, that HGH via somatomedin C (IGF-1) causes the hypertrophy of the muscles, the body viscera and the soft tissues (lips, ears, tongue, gums).This actually takes place under higher doses of somatropin (>8IU/day). Viscera (stomach, small and large intestine, kidney) have a large number of receptors IGF-1, which will lead to them inflating. This effect is not immediate, it depends on the dose and time. Therefore the abuse of r-HGH for an extended period of time creates the extrusion of the abdomen.

2) Accumulation of visceral fat occurs between the organs of the abdomen and the omentum. Greater and lesser omentumare layers of peritoneum surrounding the viscera and their vessels, nerves. Omentum creates bends and sinuses between the abdominal organs (peritoneal cavity).

The accumulation of fat happens mainly because of the lipogenesis (fat storage) induced by the use of insulin that is administrated synergistically with the HGH. Both act synergistically and the regulate glucose metabolism. Since somatropin raises serum glucose (through gluconeogenesis in liver) and insulin lowers serum glucose (and activate glycogen synthase enzyme in liver), they apparently have opposite effects on the metabolism of carbohydrates. Therefore, HGH causes hyperglycemia and the release of hepatic glycogen in blood.

This is however something thatformer chemist of BALCO & Ketosports,Patrick Arnold refuses.He supports that after the closure of epipheseal plates,hyperplastic phenomena don't occur at least in skeletal-contractile-sriated muscle tissue.

On the other hand, insulin leads to hypoglycemia and enhances formation of liver and muscle glycogen. Insulin resistance is the decrease in body's ability to respond properly to the metabolism of insulin and glucose, leading to a vicious circle of hyperglycemia, hyperinsulinemia and eventually the establishment of DM2 (non insulin dependent).

As it is known, the chronic use of r-HGHdecreases insulin sensitivity, resulting in a growing need of insulin that eventually will exceed the body's ability to properly regulate it. On that case, drugs reducing insulin resistance are required (metformin). Chromium picolinate, alpha lipoic acid and vanadyl sulphate are among the supplements that improve insulin sensitivity. While the lipolytic-fat burning action of growth hormone is generally strong enough to counteract the negative effects of insulin resistance in the fatty subcutaneous cells, it does not have the same positive effect on the visceral fat depots.

(HGH tends to reduce the natural production of thyroxin)

This occurs because it favors convertion of thyroxine to triodothyronine (T4=>T3).

The extent, to which the combination of HGH and insulin will lead to abdominal distension, differs from person to person. Factors such as the type of diet, the cardiovascular exercise, the frequency of weight lifting, the type of insulin used and the supplements can affect the sensitivity and therefore the likelihood of developing visceral fat.

3) Insulin interferes with the electrolyte balance increasing the retention of water and sodium, therefore leading to edema and swelling of tissues. This water retention occurs not only in the subcutaneous, but on the whole body as well, which is why

many people hold water in the abdomen after the injection, especially with the regular use of insulin.

4) The consumption of large portions of food is another factor of stomach distention. Therefore, the larger amounts of food consumed, the more difficult the digestion is, resulting in the distention of the intestine.

5) The chronic use of AAS in tablet form (17 alkylated) lowers and modifies the operation of the normal intestinal flora. This change disrupts the normal bowel function and causes constipation, overproduction of gas and distension of the intestine. The use of lactobacillus acidophilus probiotic bacteria as a supplement, or the consumption of kefir and organic yogurtcould be of great value.

6) Digestive disorders such gluten sensitivity and lactose intolerance that lead to the overproduction of gas in the intestine.

7) The excessive intake of red meat and the inadequate fiber intake burdens the colon, which inflames because of the toxins. In order to facilitate the digestion and assimilation of the gastrointestinal tract, it is necessary to consume vegetables and fruit that are rich in fiber every day, since that facilitates the intestinal peristalsis, prevents constipation and bowel distension.

8) The weakening of the transverse abdominal muscle plays also an essential role. The transverse abdominal muscle originates from the lumbar fascia, the last six sides, the iliac crest, the inguinal ligament and ends at white line with its denervation. It is located beneath the medial oblique and rectus abdominis muscle. The action of the transverse abdominis helps to control the body's stability, the cornering and bending of the trunk, the support of the abdominal wall and the production of intra-abdominal pressure. The transverse abdominal muscle

twitches before the other muscles of the body do, and creates the base of the body movement.Its contraction creates a rigid cylinder because of its location and its crown shape mobilizes the thoracolumbar fascia; thus creating the conditions for the increase of the intra-abdominal pressure. It acts basically like a belt around your waist, holding the truck. Relaxation of the transverse abdominis could be the result of the technique of many exercises with a large increase of intra-abdominal pressure (squats, deadlifts, leg press, lunges), leading to abdominal distension.

PEPTIDES (Secretagogues)

Secretagogues-peptides are widely used in recent years. They are composed of specific fragments of amino acids and basically they boost endogenous growth hormone production and secretion from hypophysis (GHRH).

Peptides are cheaper in the market, because they are partially growth hormone, as promoters of it. Each peptide has a specified unique sequence of amino acids and metabolic activity, thereby.

Sermorelin consists of 29 amino acids and is a well known peptide, used against growth hormone deficiency.

GH fragments are synthetic form of Ghrelin and stimulate appetite-hunger. Somatomedin C, or insulin like growth factor (IGF-1) is a 70 amino acid peptide that antagonizes the natural (endogenous) secretion of somatropin (GH) and has similar action on the metabolism of carbohydrates and fats.

On the other hand, somatostatin (GHRIH) is the inhibitor peptide of somatropin's secretion, blocking essentially the secretion of GHRH. Somatostatin (naturally released from pancreas) is administrated in cases of pituitary adenoma, in order to slow down excessive growth process and avoid gigantism.

Myostatin is a protein-peptide that hinders muscle growth, and so its inhibitor (MYOi) is also a powerful anabolic peptide. Folistatin (FST) is administrated medically in atrophic cardiomyopathy and has regenerative properties for the myocardium. As well as in idiopathic states accompanied with muscle cachexia in cancer, or muscular dystrophy, myositis (skeletal muscle inflammation), or in Duchenne Muscular Dystrophy, for example.

Researches of the New York University showed that the exogenous administration of somatropin (HGH) had a negative effect on the values of myostatin (MYO), a peptide that blocks muscle growth.

In medicine, they have been tested experimentally in acquired immunodeficiency syndrome (AIDS – HIV infection), Duchenne Muscular Dystrophy, metabolic diseases (treatment of type 2 diabetes, Cushing's syndrome) and against aging through cellular regeneration.

INSULIN AND SOMATOMEDIN C (INSULIN & IGF-1)

Insulin is one of three anabolic hormones, but actually it is a metabolic hormone produced by the islets of Langerhans in the pancreas.

It takes part in the metabolism of simple and complex carbohydrates, fats and proteins. Therefore it has a fundamental role in cellular nourishment. Its purpose is to lower blood glucose, when it increases after a meal. The property of insulin to carry all the nutrients into the muscle cell, i.e. amino acids, starch, sugars, fats, vitamins, minerals, creatine, is one of the greatest anabolic benefits for an athlete. However, insulin also regulates protein synthesis through mTOR stimulation. Its disadvantage is lipogenesis-fat store, via the lipoprotein lipase enzyme, which makes it forbidden for periods of cutting. It gives the body a feeling and an image of being "full and jacked". The muscles contract and pump better, veins increase vascularity.

The risk of a hypoglycemic episode is always possible; therefore it is advisable to eat first and then administer it, subcutaneously. A drink of simple carbohydrates (glucose, dextrose, maltodextrin) can be lifesaving at a serious sugar drop. Insulin's prolonged usage causes drowsiness and a lethargic condition.

Slow-release insulin can become fatal, under certain conditions. Slow release insulin bears the risk of a hypoglycemic episode during sleep, which can lead to a hypoglycemic coma and brain death.

On the contrary, fast-acting insulin is ideal for post training. This is actually based on the theory of the "anabolic window", when muscles absorb and utilize in maximum capacity for an hour after exercise. Besides, insulin blocks cortisol, which comes out post training as anti-inflammatory hormone and in case it's not controlled, it "cannibalizes" muscles tissue.

Insulin in combination with growth hormone-somatropin and testosterone is the ultimate gaining stack. The recommended safe dose is: one (1) IU per ten (10) kilograms of bodyweight. So an athlete whose weight is a hundred (100) kilograms, should use: ten (10)IU in total, divided in two doses preferably (breakfast and post training). The amount of carbohydrates for every ten (10)IU is 100gr of simple and complex form.

Insulin's administration does not enhance the insulin resistance and does not promote the creation of diabetes mellitus. On the contrary, it helps pancreas not to get fatigued.Insulin use will ensure that glycemia & insulin resistance coming from GH use,will be compensated,thus DM2 wont be an issue. Moreover,insulin combined to GH will make liver to release more efficiently IGF1.

Insulin like growth factor-somatomedin C (IGF-1) is a peptide consisting of 70 amino acids produced in the liver, which has a similar action as insulin on the metabolism of carbohydrates.Therefore, it promotes lipogenesis-fat storage.IGF-1 has a regenerative property on connective tissues, cartilage and muscle tissues as well. Hence, it promotes chondroblastic activity.

IGF1 has a half life of 20min, while IGFRL3 is a prolonged time released somatomedin C. IGF1 is the peptide released from liver,under exogenous use of somatotropin (HGH). Also under the presence of insulin released from pancreas,IGF1 is also released from liver.

Somatomedin C, when used exogenously, inhibits the secretion of somatropin (HGH, growth hormone), through GHRIH (somatostatin) from the pancreatic gland.

A high caloric meal increases IGF-1 concentration, while fasting reduces it.IGF-1 can be administrated intramuscularly, for instance quads, deltoids, preferable post workout at the trained muscle groups.

Metformin (Glucophage), the most widely used medication for diabetes mellitus type II taken per os to avoid insulin resistance effects.Metformin does not interfere with insulin's release from pancreas. On the contrary, it makes cellular receptors more sensitive to insulin, thus lowering insulin resistance and decreases glucose production by the liver,by inhibiting gluconeogenesis.Therefore, metformin has a beneficial impact on many components of the metabolic syndrome and diabetes mellitus type II (non insulin dependent).The action of metformin occurs only with the presence of insulin (endogenous or exogenous).

Metformin's main effect is to decrease glucose by:

-   enhancing the action of insulin in the liver primarily by suppressing hepatic glucogenesis.
-   increasing glucose intake by the muscle tissue
-   increasing glucose metabolism on gut level

However, the most serious potential side effect of metformin use isdiabetic ketoacidosis. Metformin has also been reported to decrease the blood levels of thyroid-stimulating hormone (TSH) in people with hypothyroidism.

The combination of vanadyl sulfate, alpha lipoic acid and chromium picolinate assists as glucose and insulin stabilizers.An athlete using insulin can absorb large amounts of carbohydrates and proteins per meal, leading to remarkable muscle glycogen synthesis (through glycogen synthase enzyme).Carbohydrates promote vascularity, as a result of the hypertonic environment (higher osmolality), which draws water into the venous system.

Recent studies report that increases in circulating IGF-1 levels are associated with a significantly increased risk for cancer development (prostate, colorectal, breast cancer, melanoma). Interestingly, an elevated incidence of tumors is observed also in acromegalic patients, who have elevated IGF-1 levels.Therefore, factors that promote IGF-1 hypersecretion could be linked with carcinogenesis.

These are:

- abuse of somatropin (HGH >8 IU/24h)

- hyper secretion of insulin from pancreas, followed by release of IGF-1 from the liver, as a response to a high caloric meal. Collectively, low-calorie diet and endurance exercise, which lowers insulin levels, modulate metabolic factors and reduce cancer risk.

The mechanisms responsible for the beneficial effects of calorie restriction theory on cancer prevention include:

- decreased production of growth factors and anabolic hormones (HGH, IGF-1, insulin, sex steroids)

-decreased plasma concentrations of inflammatory cytokines (IL-6, TNF) and prostaglandins (PGs).

TESTOSTERONE

It is the main androgen, the hormone that separates children from men. It was manufactured right before World War II (1935) by Germans, who received the Nobel Prize later (1939). Nazis used it extensively in order to sustain injuries and malnutrition, while aggressiveness was the main drawback.

Testosterone is produced during adolescence by the Leydig cells of testicles, being responsible for the male secondary sexualcharacteristics.These include increase of the testicular size and scrotum (nut sack), hoarseness, hirsutism, alopecia (MPB), aggression and increase of libido-sex drive.

Testosterone's effect on skeletal-striated-contractile muscles is based on hypertrophy.This is something achieved by water and electrolyte retention, leading to edema.The swelling caused by sodium and water retention in the cytoplasm-sarcoplasm, is most likely due to corticosteroids and their main representative, aldosterone. It enhances the ability of protein synthesis, through the assimilation of more animal protein (positive nitrogen balance).

Testosterone is not just anabolic, but androgenic as well.It oxidises adipose tissue, thus making the body to look harder.Testosterone becomes beneficial as an ergogenic agent during training, through the aggression stimulus that provides; especially in combination with other anabolic substances.It has a balanced ratio between androgenic and anabolic index 1:1.This is why, it is used as a basis on each steroid cycle to provide a "pseudo HPTA".

The administration of testosterone consists of 50 % of an AAS cycle. It also reduces the abdominal fat (β-oxidation), as all androgens do anyway.

Testosterone's concentration is proportional to that of somatomedin C, or Insulin like Growth Factor (IGF1), released from liver. This practically translates into their synergistic action.

Testosterone has no benefits to connective tissue growth (cartilage, ligaments, tendons), unlike growth hormone. Abuse of testosterone results in tendons' rupture, since there is no proportional development between muscles and connective tissue.

All AAS have an inverse relationship with glucocorticoids, of which the main representative is cortisol, thus they create an anabolic environment. Steroids also act as anti-inflammatory agents in certain diseases such as angioedema (stanozolol).However, the presence of glucocorticoids and cortisol has positive effect against inflammations of the musculoskeletal system. Although the injection of cortisone in the tendon bears the risk of rupture, joint pains can be suppressed only by the presence of (hydro) cortisone. Furthermore, the suppression of inflammation is a phenomenon that acts negatively on the muscle development process, since it is based on the presence of inflammation in the muscle fiber.

ARA (omega 6 MUFA) plays a significant role on that, through the increase of prostaglandins (inflammatory cytokines).The reduction of glucocorticoids during a steroid cycle lowers their anti-inflammatory effect in tendons and enhances the appearance of tendon ruptures. In case excessive muscle development is not followed by proportional connective tissue development (something that GH-IGF1 do so), detachments and ruptures of tendons and ligaments occur.

Testosterone circulates in the blood in two forms. The total testosterone (TT) which is bound to a protein, the sex hormone binding globulin (SHBG) and the free testosterone (FT) which is essentially the active form in tissues. Total testosterone is not able to penetrate the cell membrane and join the androgen receptor. The majority of testosterone is bound to the SHGB protein, which transports it into the blood serum. A very small percentage (2%) remains free-detached from sex hormone binding globulin. The higher the rate of free testosterone, the better our libido and strength. Therefore, the values of free testosterone and SHBG are inversely proportional.

As we age, the value of SHGB increases and this is also one of the reasons of andropause. Also, the increase of beta estradiol (E2) will increase the SHGB and reduce the FT. Obesity and metabolic syndrome are diseases that elevate estrogens and beta estradiol concentration.

One way to increase the value of free testosterone, is to use a synthetic form of DHT (mesterolone, drostanolone), or even danazol (used for endometriosis). This way we improve the libido, since the SHGB is reduced.

Free testosterone enters the cytoplasm of cells and joins the androgen receptor (AR). The stronger the bonding between AAS-AR is, the greater the suppression of HPTA (flouoxymesterone). Moreover, the stronger the attachment between AAS-SHGB, the more FT circulated free, therefore libido increases.

Testosterone is one of the safest injectable AAS, since it is a natural hormone that is daily produced; unlike the plethora of synthetic derivatives (AAS). It is not hepatotoxic, but has a negative effect under chronic abuse (supraphysiological doses) on the atheromatic index and the HDL/LDL ratio. It also leads to **left ventricular hypertrophy- LVH** (thickening of the left ventricular wall). This is something based on a variety of reasons:

a) Myocardium posses has androgen receptors

b) Heart muscle also consists of striated-skeletal fibers

Testosterone also increases production of sebum and skin becomes more elastic, with heavier odor. Sebum overproduction, traps microbes and infection within the hair follicles result in the form of acne (inflammation).

Testosterone's abuse results in testicular shrinkage, as a result of homeostatic cessation in endogenous testosterone production and Leydig cells.Testosterone's chronic abuse, as all androgens, may lead to psychosis and manic behavior.However, this is something depending on the genetic predisposition of each individual.

As all androgens, testosterone has a positive effect on the bone marrow, and the production of **erythropoietin** (EPO) from kidneys.Erythrocytosis and polycytemia are extreme cases of red bone marrow over stimulation.This results in the rise of hemoglobin and hematocrit.The consequence of this is a greater blood viscosity and the risk of occlusive stroke and arterial hypertension.

Testosterone can improve insulin sensitivity (or decrease insulin resistance), by improving BMI and muscle mass. Therefore, diabetic patients who use testosterone should reduce their dosage of exogenous insulin. Another issue with testosterone use is the hypertrophy of the prostate, known as benign prostatic hyperplasia (BPH), which occurs after the age of 40.

As well known, the main androgen is reduced to dihydrotestosterone (DHT), by the presence of 5a reductase enzyme. Dihydrotestosterone is a powerful androgen, a metabolite of testosterone (x 5 in vivo).This reduction takes place in different tissues, as the prostatic gland, scalp and epidermis (skin).

It is advised to those who receive testosterone replacement therapy (TRT) after the age of 40, to measure the prostate specific antigen (PSA) and undergo a digital rectal examination. It should be noticed, that the gland is also getting enlarged, under the dominance of estrogens over androgens.

Something that is mainly noticed in older people over 60.

The use of finasteride and dutasteride (inhibitors of the 5 alpha reductase enzyme) inhibit the activity of the enzyme in I and II receptors, which correspond to the prostate gland and the scalp respectively. Therefore, they deal with excessive hirsutism on the back as well as with androgenic alopecia (MPB).5a reductase inhibitors drugs are first choice medication against prostatic cancer.

However, suppression of DHT, will have a negative impact on a man's libido, gynecomastia (anti-estrogenic action of DHT), possible melancholia-moodiness (lack of DHT is associated with lower self-esteem).

DHT is an androgen with anti-estrogenic properties and five times (x5) more androgenic than testosterone (in vivo). However, there are no ergogenic benefits on muscle tissue.In local application on the nipples, it acts against gynecomastia.

Interruption during night sleep for urination (nocturia), difficulty during the start of urination and the leakage of a small amount of urine on the underwear, post urination are signs of a potential growth of the gland. Something that could be the result of prostatitis (inflammation) and elevation of PSA. In men of older age, the theory of benign hypertrophy of the prostate gland was based on dihydrotestosterone.

Metabolites of DHT are those AAS that do not aromatize, like mesterolone, methenolone, stanozolol, oxandrolone, drostanolone, oxymetholone. Finasteride, dutasteride (5 alpha reductase inhibitors) have no effect on male pattern baldness (androgenic alopecia) and benign prostatic hyperplasia. DHT derivatives have a less suppressive effect on HPTA, in less extend than the metabolites of testosterone (equipoise, fluoxymesterone).

The administration of testosterone in men over 40 has been proven to be a major anti-depressant, which contributes to antiaging. Testosterone supports the muscular system, provides a more elastic skin, enhances libido and promotes self confidence. The thoughts become more decisive, while women are attracted to men with high testosterone, through their skin odor.

Hormone replacement with testosterone (TRT) and DHEA has positive effects on reducing the abdominal fat and insulin resistance. The increase of the abdominal fat promotes the creation of the metabolic syndrome, as well as insulin resistance promotes the creation of lipogenesis (a predisposing factor of diabetes mellitus type II, non insulin dependent).

Because testosterone's biosynthesis initiates from another steroid molecule, cholesterol, it is reasonable why diets low in saturated fats will have a negative impact on its endogenous production

Modern medication such as statins lower total cholesterol and low density lipoprotein LDL. The final result would be to lower total testosterone's serum levels as well.

Biosynthesis of cholesterol is a process that takes place in the liver parenchyma. The Leydig cells of the testicles produce approximately between 7-10 mg of the hormone on a daily basis. This translates into approximately 50-70mg on a weekly basis; roughly ten to twenty times lower than the abuse of a competitive bodybuilder. Just by this fact, we understand the degree of atrophy testicles undergo. It makes sense that after years of AAS abuse, the male ends up hypogonadic for life. A crushed libido and oligospermia, along with increased body fat, low self confidence, poor muscularity and loss of muscle

Bodybuilding

endurance-strength are present.Not to neglect the negative consequences of a chronic overdose-abuse on the myocardium, the atheromatic index, the prostatic hypertrophy, polycytemia, androgenic alopecia.

Last but not least, the effects on mental health. This is the price every competitive or recreational bodybuilder has to pay eventually.

Biosynthesis of testosterone's steroid molecule

Slow esters of testosterone (enanthate, cypionate) are released gradually, reaching a peak around day four and remaining in the body for a prolonged timing (7-10 days). Aromatization is easier to occur, as a result of this longer half life.The clinical symptom of gynecomastia is an aesthetic issue, where the nipple is swollen and painful-touchy under palpation.

Enanthate and cypionate esters, release a smaller amount of active testosterone, around 70%.In contrast, fast esters (propionate, suspension) have very immediate results, with the disadvantage that they have to be administered more often.Three times a week for the propionate and on a daily basis for the water-soluble-suspension, ester-free form. They provide a greater amount of testosterone (80% and 100% respectively).Therefore, testosterone suspension is the most powerful type among injectable testosterones.Fast acting esters have a lesser chance for aromatization, as a result of their short half life into the body. They are preferably used during pre-contest preparation.

However it should be noticed, that the more estrogenic an AAS is, the greater anabolic properties it has. After all, aromatization and water retention is a fundamental biochemical environment that supports muscle growth and strength. Testosterone is converted into estrogen, by the

enzyme aromatase in the mammary gland, adipose-fat tissue, liver and brain. Obese individuals have elevated levels of (E2) beta estradiol, as a result of greater body fat percentage.

Testosterone applied in the form of a gel, increases the serum levels of dihydrotestosterone (DHT), since the skin has increased concentration of 5a reductase enzyme. The transdermal absorption of testosterone has only 10% absorbency, but the advantage of sustained release and stable blood levels, compared to the intramuscular (IM) use.Parenteral (intramuscular) type of administration acts acute into the circulation.The subcutaneous (SC) use has a delayed absorption and this is why insulin is usually administered under the skin. Somatropin (HGH) is administrated subcutaneously because of its lipolytic (fat burning) ability, that also provides a delayed absorption time. During a steroid cycle, the ration between androgens and anabolics should be (2:1). This will ensure there is no crush on libido and sexual drive.

Testosterone has the ability to suppress the production of catabolic cortisol (the main corticosteroid).This is the reason why after the end of a cycle, both cortisol and estrogens rebound and rise dramatically. As a result of it, the physique gets smooth and muscle wasting occurs (catabolism).

The use of anti-estrogenic compounds (SERMs, tamoxifen) has a negative impact on testosterone's benefits, regarding muscle growth. Tamoxifen citrate is known to suppress IGF1 in liver.On the other hand the significance of the estrogenic environment to muscle growth is fundamental.Estrogens enhance muscle glycogen synthesis, through water retention. Therefore, muscle strength and stamina is enhanced. Estrogens are known to improve steroid receptors affinity to the steroid molecules. Estrogens improve joints lubrication, by retaining water into the synovial cavity.This is something critical under off season heavy duty training. Proof that women produce testosterone,but a lesser amount than men, is the fact that older women have increased facial hair, known as hirsutism. This practically occurs after the menopause when estrogens are no longer produced.

Androgens produced by the adrenal glands and ovaries, continue their action, and therefore manifest their androgenic secondary characteristics. Androgens can act therapeutically, though, for a woman in the case of breast cancer. The estrogens are in exacerbation, so androgens (fluoxymesterone, drostanolone) act as an alternative treatment. Nowadays, under the new generation of anti-estrogens (anastrozole, letrozole, exemestane) the use of 17 alkylated hepatotoxic AAS is no longer necessary.

TESTOSTERONE, THE WONDER MEDICATION

As a doctor who follows TRT for the past five years, my belief is that TRT is ruining big pharma sales. You see, testosterone is a cheaper drug compared to other medications who treat some of the symptoms testosterone does: Insulin resistance and DM2. Anemia, arthritis, osteopenia, depression, erectile dysfunction, dyslipidemia, obesity and metabolic syndrome. Certainly each medical treatment faces potential side effects, but in every treatment we always should balance prons and cons. The point is that hypogonadic men cant live without testosterone. However they surely can live without growth hormone during andropause and GHRH deficiency. But nothing can replace the main androgen (as women are suffering in the absence of estrogens during menopause). It's a fact that the plethora of benefits TRT provides in different tissues, makes it to be considered as a wonder medicine and apparently this is not accepted by the big pharmaceutical industries. Testosterone was given a bad name throughout its abuse from bodybuilders. This is how the medical world became skeptical and deals with suspicion the main androgen. Testosterone however is a familiar hormone and not a synthetic derivative like the rest of AAS instead. It has not side effects in liver and lipids, unlike anabolic steroids do.

TESTOSTERONE'S SYNTHETIC DERIVATIVES

17 ALKYLATED AAS

17 alkylated androgenic-anabolic steroids (AAS) is a class of synthetic derivatives of testosterone, which have undergone a specific modification (methylation).This enables oral steroids to sustain the first entrance to the liver. However, this fact stresses hepatic parenchyma, thus elevating liver enzymes known as transaminases (alanine transaminase ALT/SGOT and aspartate transaminase AST/SGPT).

17 alkylated aas include:

1) stanozolol (both oral and injectable form)
2) oxymetholone
3) methandienone (there was an injectable form by Ciba)
4) oxandrolone
5) fluoxymesterone
6) methyltrienolone (M3)

They are not aromatized, except methandienone-methandrostenolone, perhaps the most widely abused AAS pill.

They are powerful anabolic agents, while during dieting period they have a strong anti-catabolic effect. They also provide necessary aggressiveness during training, especially in periods of harsh dieting.

Their main side effects include:

- distortion of atheromatic index and the lipoproteins ratio (HDL/LDL cholesterol).

The main reason for the reduction of high density lipoprotein (HDL), is the stimulation of a protein (endothelial hepatic triglyceride lipase), responsible for the transfer of HDL to the liver.

- pharmaceutical hepatitis, followed by transaminasemia (ALT/AST-SGPT/SGOT). These elevations are usually asymptomatic, transient and return to baseline levels within several weeks after cessation. Such elevations have been most closely linked to fluoxymesterone and oxymetholone.

Recently, studies demonstrated that GGT, ALP are the most distinctive enzymes (cholestatic) for the detection of hepatic dysfunction (jaundice).

Whenever we combine two or more 17 alkylated orals (stanozolol, oxymethelone, methyltrienolone, methandrostenolone), it is advisable to use them sublingually, **i.e. under the tongue**. By this method, we avoid and bypass the first entrance to liver metabolism, **the substance does not affect directly the liver and less liver strain occurs.** Instead, they are rapidly absorbed by the tiny capillary network under the tongue, thus entering circulation and bloodstream. Pharmacokinetics is more immediate this way.

Since 17 alkylated orals are responsible of atheromatic index distortion, their abuse may lead to cardiovascular disease (CVD). Moreover, blood coagulation is distorted, since clotting factors which are synthesized in the liver, are disturbed.

Bodybuilding

Prothrombin time (PT) and international normalized ratio (INR) are prolonged. It should be noted that the bleeding tendency accounts for increased risk of morbidity and mortality in AAS abusers.

<u>Methandrostenolone – methandienone</u> (Dianabol) is a derivative of methyl-testosterone. Methandienone aromatises and the administration of an anti-estrogenic agent is necessary (anastrozole-letrozole-exemestane or tamoxifen-mesterolone), in order to avoid gynecomastia, or the retention of water and lipogenesis-fat storage. The edema followed by aromatization process, is beneficial for muscle glycogen formation. This is something very important for anabolism, since strength and stamina are enhanced. Muscle are able to contract much better and look fuller, "pumped". This water retention due to estrogenic activity, lubricates synovial cavities, hence it protects the joints.

Methandienone is medically used during postoperative syndromes, when the patient is malnourished and needs immediate assimilation of nutrients and tissue regeneration. It is also very useful against muscle wasting and cachexia.

Dianabol's half life is estimated around six hours, therefore it should be administrated four times a day during the course of 24 hours.

Dianabol's use is often linked to acne and skin inflammation. This could be the result of aromatization and its moderate androgenic index.

<u>Oxymetholone</u> (Anadrol 50) is medically prescribed for aplastic anemia and it increases EPO production from kidneys. Iron absorption improves in small intestine and erythrocytosis

process improves. As a result, hemoglobin protein elevates, so does hematocrit. From chemical point of view, oxymetholone is a DHT derivative. Therefore, aromatization is something out of the question.

However, oxymetholone's metabolites have showed a great affinity for the estrogen receptors. This is something observed under estrogenic environment. When oxymetholone is administrated alone, while beta estradiol levels are relatively low, there is no particular aromatization. However, under the presence of other AAS with estrogenic activity, aromatization occurs. This explains why within a gaining cycle with testosterone, nandrolone, boldenone and methandienone, oxymetholone seems to aromatize and be able for extreme water retention. Increased blood pressure, due to sodium retention, is a common side effect of it, while often the feeling of nausea and the tendency to vomit appears. Its androgenic property leads to acne and aggressive behavior. Its half life is around nine hours, which means it should be administrated twice a day.

Oxandrolone (Anavar) is a powerful anabolic steroid pill (per os), with a more powerful anabolic index than oxymetholone comparing mg/mg. Its low androgenic index makes it preferable among females, in order to avoid the non reversible side effects of androgens (hirsutism, voice deepening, clitoris enlargement).

Oxandrolone is a derivative of dihydrotestosterone (DHT). Since there is no aromatization and considerable low androgenic activity, the suppress to HPTA is less. Adversely, it is hepatotoxic, causing elevation of the liver enzymes, known as transaminases (SGOT-AST, SGPT-ALT,). It also distorts atheromatic index and lipoprotein ratio (HDL/LDL).

Oxandrolone can increase ATP/CP production, thus making it a useful tool among explosive sports in track athletics (sprinting, jumps).

The fact it does not lead to any aromatization, water retention and edema, makes oxandrolone a favorable AAS among athletes with the weight class. Among bodybuilders, oxandrolone is highly abused during pre contest preparations, while dieting. In doses >50mg daily, it increases serum free thyroxine (FT4) and contributes to catabolism of adipose tissue and lipolysis (beta oxidation). Its half life is approximately eight hours, so it should be taken three times during the day.

The hepatotoxic fluoxymesterone (Halotestin) is a testosterone's derivative, highly androgenic (eight times more than testosterone) and anabolic as well. It is ideal for sports, dealing with weight class (boxing, wrestling, bodybuilding, and weightlifting). Halotestin provides enormous increase in strength, which in combination with a low carb diet, offers muscle density and thickness. Fluoxymesterone's supreme androgenicity favors prostate enlargement-hypertrophy, acne, androgenic alopecia, hirsuitism, erythocytosis plus beta oxidation of adipose tissue and aggressiveness.

As a 17 alkylated AAS, causes distortion of atheromatic index and the lipoproteins ratio (HDL/LDL cholesterol) and pharmaceutical hepatitis. Furthermore, it increases systemic blood pressure and along with the adverse side effect on lipoproteins, increases the risk of cardiovascular disease and myocardial infarction.

Fluoxymesterone is speculated to cause neurotoxicity, affecting the central nervous system. Episodes of insomnia, aggression (physical and verbal), irritability, anxiety, neurosis, mood swings-emotional instability, hypomania and depression have been associated with this substance abuse.

However, these effects are correlated to the severity of abuse in terms of dosage and time period, the psychiatric background of the individual, the simultaneous use of different neurotoxic chemicals (ethanol or narcotics).

As a testosterone's derivative and as a highly androgenic agent, fluoxymesterone is highly suppressive to HPTA. Fluoxymesterone shouldn't be abused for longer than four weeks, along with proper supplementation (milk thisle, NAC, glutathione).

Since it does not aromatizeand convert to estrogen, Halotestin is a preferable drug during precontest preparation, prolonged dieting. Although it is considered to be highly anabolic, the fact it does not lead to any form of edema, makes this steroid a poor bulking agent.However, it is more likely to be used during off season timing, for gaining strength purposes, or among powerlifters, Olympic weightlifters.

Methyltrienolone (M3) is a trenbolone's derivative,perhaps the most hepatotoxic oral among the 17 alkylated AAS. It was initially medically used against advanced breast cancer, as an alternative treatment to the rise of estrogens. It has a similarity to trenbolone, with an enormous androgenic/anabolic ratio.Its effectiveness is so high, that it requires minimum doses of 0,5-1mg. M3 does not convert to estrogens, therefore there is no aromatization process. As a result, methyltrienolone is an ideal steroid during pre contest preparation and sports dealing with weight categories (wrestling, weightlifting, boxing, and bodybuilding).

The extreme liver toxicity involves pharmaceutical hepatitis, where liver transaminases are elevated (>100) and cholestasis, where serumelevations of cholestatic markers such as ALP, γGT, bilirubin-direct/indirect, are present. Methyltrienolone also distorts the atheromatic index (HDL/LDL) and liver lipoproteins ratio, increasing the risk of cardiovascular disease and myocardial infarction.

The injectable (parenteral) form of stanozolol (Winstrol depot) is less toxic to the liver, since it avoids the first hepatic entrance and enters directly into circulation. It is a suspension and usually painful, when administrated intramuscularly.

Its half life is around 24 hours, which practically means that has to be daily administrated, preferably an hour before workout.

Injectable stanozolol could lead to local inflammation accompanied with fever, while in extreme cases, it may lead to an intramuscular abscess.

Generally, suspension steroids are more likely to develop microbes compared to oily injections.Contamination is something easier to occur in suspensions (stanozolol, testosterone, trenbolone base).Unlike other oily injectable steroids, stanozolol tends to remove water from the joints.This is something based on the aldosterone inhibition (mineral corticosteroid).Therefore, stanozolol is an anabolic steroid that does not lead to any water retention.Consequently, joints aren't lubricated and synovial cavities dry and literally get "toasted".Stanozolol should not be combined with accutane (retinoic acid), a drug against cystic acne. Accutane dries mucous membranes, causing dry skin and reduction of sebum production. This effect combined with the drain of water from synovial space, leads to tendons and ligaments rupture.

Stanozolol suspension has a milky-whitish appearance, with a relatively low concentration (50mg/ml). As all anabolic steroids, stanozolol is capable for tissue growth and repair. It also has the ability for collagen fibers connective tissue synthesis. Its authenticity is checked, after we let an ampoule vertically for about an hour. Afterwards, we should observe the water's and the sediment's ratios (1/1). If water's percentage is superior to the white powder, then it is highly possible to be under dosed. By that, we refer to the suspension's concentration. This case scenario seems better, related to a faked steroid, where the supposed substance does not exist. However, that could be also related to the size of particles within the suspension. Usually, expensive compounds are faked by cheaper ones. For instance, methenolone (Primobolan) and oxandrolone (Anavar) are faked by nandrolone (Decadurabolin) and methandienone (Dianabol).

Winstrol depot should be preferably administrated one hour prior to the gym, since the absorbability is immediate (100%), as with all suspensions.

OTHER AAS

(nandrolone, methenolone, boldenone, mesterolone, drostanolone, trenbolone)

Two of the safest injectable AAS for the liver are nandrolone (Decadurabolin-Organon, class of 19nortestosterone derivatives) and the enanthate form of Methenolone (Primobolan Depot-Bayer/Schering).

Methenolone is a mild non aromatized anabolic steroid with a low androgenic index.It is considered as a derivative of dihydrotestosterone (DHT). As a result, it does not lead to any water retention or gynecomastia (E2- beta estradiol elevation).Therefore, methenolone enanthate-acetate are ideal during cutting sessions (precontest preparation). Its low androgenicity makes it preferable for female use. The injectable form of methenolone consists of enanthate ester for depot intramuscular injection.

It has a lower anabolic index compared to nandrolone and lower androgenicity than testosterone.It takes about four weeks in order to observe any positive effects concerning muscle strength.

Methenolone tablet for oral administration is of immediate release (methenolone acetate).Methenolone acetate does not present hepatotoxicity (non-17 alkylated). Therefore it does not elevate liver enzymes (AST/ALT). Furthermore, it has a slight negative impact on atheromatic index and lipids (HDL/LDL).

Nandrolone is an anabolic steroid more anabolic than methenolone, which promotes strength and lean muscle mass gain. The drug has a positive effect in joints and their lubrication.It stimulates aldosterone from the kidneys, leading to sodium retention and edema. Moreover, it enhances calcium reabsorption in renal tubules. The positive influence in calcium metabolism makes nandrolone an ideal drug against osteopenia and osteoporotic fractures. Nandrolone decaonate (Deca-Durabolin) lubricates synovial cavities, thus suppressing pain under moderation dosage (50mg/week). On the other hand, this can be dangerous, since the improvement of pain eases the impact of heavy weights and forces the athlete for a heavy work out. At this point, it is highly possible for musculoskeletal injuries such as tendon and muscle ruptures to occur.

Nandrolone significantly suppresses the hypothalamic pituitary testicular axis and crushes on libido. 19 nortestosterone derivatives are linked to progestational activity and production of prolactin, a hormone which augments gynecomastia and body fat gain.

However, it should be noted that 19nor anabolic androgenic steroids (AAS) lead to prolactinemia, in the presence of elevated estrogens (E2-beta estradiol). If E2 level is low, then prolactine does not rise enough, to suppress testosterone. The use of dopamine agonists (bromocriptine, cabergoline) seems obligatory in order to suppress prolactine's serum levels. Consequently, libido is improved.

Nandrolone has negative effects on serum lipids (reduction of high density lipoprotein HDL-, increase in low density lipoprotein LDL- and total cholesterol), which are dose and time dependant.

The drug is also responsible for arterial calcification and stable plaque formation, all potentially increasing the risk of cardiovascular disease. It may also lead to kidney stones formation, in the presence of impaired hydration, excessive protein and salt intake.

Nandrolone is aromatized relatively easily at doses above 400mg per week. Nandrolone decaonate (Deca-Durabolin) is a long time release AAS, where almost 60% of the substance is utilized. On the contrary, the phenylpropionate ester has a faster half life of immediate release (80%).

Boldenone (Equipose) is a veterinary injectable anabolic steroid, a derivative of testosterone.It exhibits strong androgenic and anabolic properties. It is moderately aromatised to beta estradiol (E2) compared to nandrolone, therefore leading to less water retention. However estrogenic side effects such as gynecomastia and body fat gain are noticed in doses above 400 mg per week. As a derivative of testosterone, it suppresses the hypothalamic-pituitary-gonadal axis to a greater degree, compared to the DHT derivatives.

It stimulates appetite, vascularity and red bone marrow, increasing red blood cell production (erythropoietic effect). As a result, boldenone increases the values of hematocrit (Htc), hemoglobin (Hgb) and myoglobin too. It is a slow sustained release compound (undecylenate ester), which requires more than four weeks in order someone to observe any positive feedback. VeterinaryEquipose is available in 50mg/ml. However a denser variety of boldenone is also available by underground laboratories at 200mg/ml.

Mesterolone(Proviron) is a synthetic form of diydroxytestosterone (DHT).It has a mild anti-estrogenic and androgenic action. Mesterolone improves body composition, through beta oxidation of fatty acids. It improves dramatically libido, since it binds strongly with the sex hormone binding globulin (SHBG).Therefore, it allows free testosterone (FT) to circulate. DHT as a substance is considered to be five times more androgenic than testosterone. However DHT has no positive effect on skeletal muscle and growth.

Mesterolone, along with drostanolone and SERMs, could become an alternative form of anti-estrogenic treatment within a cycle, in order to avoid the side effects of potent aromatase inhibitors. It is the only pharmaceutical grade AAS pill, which is not 17- alkylated. Therefore, hepatotoxicity is unlikely.

Mesterolone affects benign prostate hyperplasia (BPH), male pattern hair loss (MPB-androgenic alopecia) and body/facial hair growth. In high doses it is suppressive to hypothalamic-pituitary-testicular axis (HPTA).As all AAS, mesterolone has negative effects on serum lipids (reduction of high density lipoprotein-HDL-, increase in low density lipoprotein-LDL- and total cholesterol), which are dose and time dependant. 5a reductase inhibitors (finasteride, dutasteride) effect mesterolone's metabolism.

The drugs that are used for bulking purposes (testosterone enanthate-cypionate, methandrostenolone, oxymetholone, nandrolone,equipose) lead to edema-swelling of tissues, as a result of water and sodium retention. This has an adverse effect on blood pressure, with an increase of both its systolic and diastolic values. It is advisable during that period to reduce the consumption of table salt and drink plenty of water, low insodium.Also do not neglect the significance of potassium, which is known to act competitively in the Na/K pump cell membrane.

Drostanolone (Masteron) is medically prescribed as an anti-estrogenic therapy for the treatment of advanced inoperable breast cancer in postmenopausal women. It was originally manufactured under pharmaceutical production by

Lilly/Syntex during the late 1960s. It was withdrawn in late 90s in Belgium.

The drug is an injectable AAS derived from dihydrotestosterone (DHT). It presents milder androgenicity than testosterone and higher anabolic index, similar to that of nandrolone. Drostanolone has anti-estrogenic properties, since there is no aromatisation (conversion to estrogen) and water retention; therefore, the drug usually replaces testosterone.

It is advisable to be used during the end of a precontest preparation, when physique has low body fat percentage and looks "harder". Masteron is available in fast-propionate ester, thus it should be administrated every other day or so. It can be stacked perfectly well with trenbolone and fluoxymesterone during the last two weeks before a contest. Both drostanolone and mesterolone (injectable and per os forms DHT), can be alternative anti-estrogenic options combined with tamoxifen citrate (SERM).This plan avoids the use of powerful aromatase inhibitors, which can become harmful to serum lipids (HDL, LDL, cholesterol) and lipoprotein ratio (HDL/LDL). Drostanolone affects the metabolism of 5a reductase and production of DHT.

Therefore, hypertrophy of the prostate gland (BPH) or male alopecia (MPB) are more likely to occur.5 a reductase inhibitors (finasteride, dutasteride) effect drostanolone's metabolism.

<u>Trenbolone</u> is a 19-nortestosterone derivative with a chemical structure resembling nandrolone.It is of high androgenicity and anabolic activity (about five times higher that testosterone), ideal during precontest preparation and dieting. Trenbolone has a positive effect on fat burning and catabolism of adipose tissue (beta oxidation).It is a progestin, leading to progestational activity which raises prolactine in the presence of estrogens.

Trenbolone is available in slow, intermediate and fast acting injectable esters (enanthate, hexahydrobenzylcarbonate, acetate). Acetate and enanthate forms are not for human use, as they are used in veterinary medicine for cattles.

Only Parabolan(trenbolonehexahydrobenzylcarbonate) was available for human use manufactured by Negma pharmaceutical company in the 80's and was discontinued in 1997.Trenbolone enanthate (slow ester) releases 70% of the substance, while the intermediate 80%.Fast ester has a short half life and highest degree of assimilation, even higher than of testosterone propionate (90%).However, for the past five years there has been available in the market, a suspension form (trenbolone base 50mg) with an acute absorbability (100%) and a half life of 24h.

Trenbolone presents negative impact on serum lipids [decreased high density lipoprotein (HDL), increased low density lipoprotein (LDL) and triglycerides] and may increase systemic blood pressure. All these factors are associated with an increased risk of atherosclerosis and coronary heart disease. As a progestational steroid, it raises prolactine. Apart from aesthetic issues of gynecomastia, prolactinemia also affects libido and sexual drive. Dopamine agonists (bromocriptine, cabergoline) should be used along with trenbolone, in order to improve libido, by lowering serum prolactine.

Androgenic side effects include acne, body/facial hair growth, male pattern hair loss (MPB-androgenic alopecia) and benign prostate hyperplasia (BPH). Studies have shown that trenbolone plays critical roles in neurodegeneration and apoptosis in hippocampus-amygdala. Hippocampus is a certain area in mesencephalon, belonging to the limbic system, associated with behavior. Abuse can develop episodes of insomnia, aggression (physical and verbal), irritability, anxiety, neurosis, mood

Bodybuilding

swings-emotional instability, manic episodes, depression and rarely psychosis-misconceptions.

The authenticity of the fast ester is noticed by the appearance of the typical "tren cough" soon after the intramuscular injection. High concentration of trenbolone acetate, along with the presence of benzolium (alcohol with distinctive smell) can directly irritate lung tissue. These substances cause an asthmatic crisis with bronchospasm and symptoms of paroxysmal coughing, wheezing, rapid breathing or chest pressure. Immediate use of bronchodilators such as inhaled salbutamol is necessary. Another factor that is responsible for "tren cough" is the introduction of a small amount of oil into small blood vessels, or the lymphatic system during intramuscular injection.

Trenbolone is known to cause a reduction of aerobic capacity. Based on the fact that it is a "cortisol crusher", trenbolone stimulates inflammation. Therefore, inflammatory cytokines-prostaglandins (PG's) in the respiratory system trigger bronchospasm and infections, leading to poor respiratory capacity (VO2max). On the other hand, the "cortisol crush" makes trenbolone highly anabolic. As known, cortisol (glucocorticoid) is considered to be a muscle catabolic hormone. Since cortisol induces hyperglycemia through gluconeogenesis, trenbolone's use will lead to hypoglycemia.

Trenbolone is considered as a precontest anabolic steroid, since there is no water retention and edema effect, based on aldosterone's and cortisol's inhibition from the kidneys. On the contrary, cortisol's crush leads to joint discomfort, since cortisol is known to mask pain and sooth joint aches. People with increased muscle mass (BMI>30) also have elevated levels of creatinine, as the striated-skeletal muscles have more creatine, even when it is not exogenously obtained in the form of mono-hydrate powder. Trenbolone combined with creatine and diuretics can cause renal strain and elevation of indexes.Increased blood pressure derived from the action of clenbuterol hydrochloride (beta2-agonists), can potentially cause sclerosis of the renal tubules because of extensive vasoconstriction, which leads to an increase of blood pressure.

As it is known some androgenic anabolic steroids are ideal for combating osteoporosis (nandrolone). This is because growing muscles can be adhered better to the bones and those gain higher density as a reaction. The other reason is because the AAS cause retention of sodium and calcium, which strengthens the bones and causes undesirable swelling. Unfortunately, the hypercalcemia leads to nephrolithiasis, situations that lead to complications in the urinary tract. Moreover it may lead to endothelium calcifucation of coronary and carotid arteries than might occlude and lower blood supply to heart and brain.

PHARMAKOKINETICS OF AAS

STEROIDS WITH THE HIGHEST ANDROGENIC INDEX
1) methyltrienolone (6000)
2) fluoxymesterone (800)
3) trenbolone (500)

STEROIDS WITH THE LOWEST ANDROGENIC INDEX
1) oxandrolone (24)
2) stanozolol (30)
3) nandrolone (37)
4) oxymetholone (45)
5) boldenone (50)
6) methenolone (57)

SLOW RELEASE INJECTABLE AAS
1) testosterone enanthate
2) testosterone cypionate
3) testosterone undecaonate (per os)
4) testosterone decaonate
5) methenolone enanthate (DHT derivative)

6) trenbolone enanthate (19nor derivative)

7) nandrolone undecaonate (19nor derivative)

8) boldenone undecyclate (testosterone derivative)

IMMEDIATE RELEASE INJECTABLE AAS

1) stanozolol suspension (DHT derivative)

2) nandrolone phenylpropionate (19nor derivative)

3) testosterone propionate

4) testosterone suspension

5) drostenolone propionate (DHT synthetic)

6) trenbolone acetate (19nor derivative)

7) trenbolone suspension-base (19nor derivative)

AROMATIZED AAS

1) testosterone

2) oxymetholone? (DHT derivative)

3) methyldrostenolone (methyltestosterone derivative)

4) methyltestosterone (testosterone derivative)

5) nandrolone undecaonate (19nor derivative)

NON AROMATIZED AAS (DHT derivatives)

1) stanozolol

2) oxandrolone

3) mesterolone

4) methenolone

5) fluoxymesterone (testosterone derivative)

6) trenbolone acetate (19nor derivative)

7) drostenolone propionate (DHT synthetic)

The higher androgenic index a steroid has, the more effective is for beta oxidation-lipolysis of the subcutaneous tissue, leading to muscle hardness. On the other hand, there is a higher reduction rate to dihydrotestosterone, leading to andogenic side effects such as benign prostatic hyperplasia, male pattern baldness-androgenic alopecia, acne, oily skin, body/facial hair growth, aggressive behavior, as well as erythrocytosis.

Anabolic steroids having a lower androgenic index than testosterone can cause a positive nitrogen balance-tissue anabolism and act against catabolism. Furthermore, the androgenic side effects (acne, hirsutism, neuropsychiatric disorders, prostate enlargement, male-pattern baldness, suppression of the hypothalamic pituitary testicular axis, neuropsychiatric disorders) will be less, but always are dose and time dependent.

AUTHENTICITY OF AAS

As a competitive bodybuilder, I have to admit, I was quite skeptical to the point of suspicion, regarding how legit were AAS. My main concern was regarding the substance used, while to a lesser degree, dosage. Therefore, I mainly was focusing on pharmaceuticals, officially approved by the drug association of each country.

The use of injectable steroids in single ampoules is preferable, since it's harder to be faked. The construction cost of a single ampoule is way higher related to a bottle of 10ml. As a result, a faked 10ml bottle would bring higher profits to the manufacturers. Sterilization conditions are also safer, in disposable ampoules.

There are three main classes of AAS in the market:

1) the limited genuine and safe medicinal products, being authorized by the drug association of the particular country,

2) the underground (non-pharmaceutical) laboratories which replicate almost all substances that no longer exist in the global pharmaceutical market,

3) the counterfeits which are identical copies of original pharmaceuticals.

The problem with counterfeits & undergrounds is not just being under dosed relative to the labeled, but the possibility of containing a different substance.For instance, nandrolone decaonate (Decadurabolin) is usually the faked steroid, instead of methenolone enanthate (Primobolan); or metandienone (Dianabol), instead of oxandrolone (Anavar).

Regarding the credibility of a particular substance, we could identify from specific blood tests if the particular AAS is original; DHT derivatives (oxandrolone, methenolone, stanozolol) and synthetic forms of DHT (drostanolone, mesterolone).

We know that DHT derivatives do not aromatize. Therefore, if beta estradiol (E2) is elevated, then we assume that the particular AAS is faked.

So instead of oxandrolone, it could have being methandrostenolone, or instead of methenolone, nandrolone could be a possible case.

In case stanozolol suspension aromatizes, then most likely it is testosterone suspension solution.

In some cases nandrolone elevates prolactin, especially when and if E2 is already high enough. Therefore, if someone uses boldenone and prolactin is elevated, then it is possible that equipose is faked by Deca-Durabolin. Other indications include the shutdown of HPTA in every AAS use and dramatic elevation of TT, FT.

The disadvantage of this method is that each substance has to be measured separately. Stacking different AAS would not help to clarify if the chemical is original.

Another issue that should be concerned is the presence of second class oils and heavy metals, which accumulate in the body. There are specific criteria for notification and identification of false AAS, which have to do with specific evidence-marks on their paper and glass packaging.

INTRAMUSCULAR ABSCESS

Occasionally, bodybuilders develop intramuscular abscesses, septic and sterile,as a result of deep IM shots. The main difference between them is that the former develops the clinical symptoms of inflammation and deals with infection, while the later deals with hard lumps of oily solutions. In the long term, they get calcified and turn into scar tissue.

Septic abscess is a result of contaminated injectable steroid solutions or non-sterile injection techniques (needle sharing, reusing needles and syringes). Common areas include the buttocks (gluteus maximus), shoulders (deltoid), chest (pectoralis), calves (gastrognemius).

Oily androgenic anabolic steroids (AAS) solutions usually aren't contaminated, since the oily solution is a hostile environment for bacterial growth. On the contrary, water based suspension solutions, such as stanozolol, testosterone and recently trenbolone base are among the riskier injectables. Bacteria are likely to get cultivated in such solutions and as a result, inflammation occurs. Thigh abscesses, pectoral and deltoid abscess have been reported in bodybuilders using 'spot shots' or 'site locations', which are local injections into a specific muscle, believed to increase isolated muscle growth. Gluteal abscesses have also occurred in contaminated products. Administration of large volumes of testosterone esters in one injection (up to 5 mL) is common, exposing an individual to sterile abscess formation, where a pathogenic organism cannot be found.

Reported infections associated with AAS injection include abscesses attributable to Staphylococcus, Streptococcus, Pseudomonas and atypical Mycobacteria. The basic sings of inflammation process include: 1) local swelling-edema, 2) erythema, 3) elevated temperature/ pyrexia and 4) pain. All of these symptoms take place due to the increased blood flow, since macrophages and neutrophils are among the white blood cells responsible for phagocytosis of microorganisms. An abscess is a defensive reaction of the tissue to prevent the spread of infectious materials to other parts of the body.

Besides clinical and laboratory findings [leukocytosis with increased neutrophils, elevated erythrocyte sedimentation rate (ESR) and C-reactive protein (CRP)], a useful laboratory examination that reveals the existence of intramuscular abscess, is the Magnetic Resonance Image (MRI), ideal for the soft tissues (muscles, joints, ligaments, tendons).

Abscesses should not be squeezed by the person concerned. If the abscess burst under the skin and the bacteria spread through the blood circulation into the body, it can result in a life-threatening blood infection such as sepsis. Sepsis symptoms include general malaise, fever, chills, nausea, vomiting, diarrhea, tachypnea, and confusion. Sepsis always requires hospitalization.

Initially the steroid user should avoid injecting into the inflamed area, while rotating the injection spots. Quitting from injections at least for one week, will give some time for the immune system to suppress the intramuscular inflammation. The use of nonsteroidal anti-inflammatory drugs-NSAIDs (sodium diclophenac, nimesulide) could provide some aid in first place and fight discomfort. Furthermore, hypertonic solution based on aluminum, provides pain relief when applied locally with a wet towel for about 10 minutes 4 times daily. A pharmaceutical medication that has a significant role in order to prevent further edema is the rerapeptase drug. This drug is widely used in several cases that include septic, or non septic inflammation, where excessive swelling is present. Finally, the danaparoid sodium cream is a helpful material, able to suppress edema, thus providing a relief feeling. However, sometimes inflammation process is more severe and complicated and pus develops in the intramuscular abscess. Pus contains dead white blood cells, trying to control the inflammation. In the beginning, an intramuscular infection is reddish and sort of hard in touch. Later, as the inflammation proceeds and pus is gathered, it becomes softer. Usually surgeons find this a warning sign, where surgical incision and drainage is obligatory. The surgeon cuts the skin and fat beneath with a scalpel, entering the inflamed muscle. This will give the opportunity for the drug (oily) solution and pus to leave the contaminated area, which has to be excessively cleaned afterwards. As soon as the pus has drained, the surgeon will insert some packing into the remaining cavity to minimize any bleeding and keep it open for 24–48 hours. As the scar heals, the patient can expect to be out of the gym for weeks. If it is a deeper abscess, the surgeon may insert a drainage tube. Drainage is maintained for several days to help prevent the abscess from reforming.

Microbiological culture of biologic samples from the wound is performed by the biopathologist and according to the antibiogram, a proper medication shall be prescribed. In most cases, the physician supplies a combination of different antibiotics, including treatment of aerobic and anaerobic bacteria. In those cases an anti-staphylococcus antibiotic (flucloxacillin, dicloxacillin) or amoxicillin- clavulanic acid is given. Alternative antibiotics effective against community-acquired methicillin-resistant Staphylococcus aureus (MRSA) often include clindamycin, doxycycline, minocycline, and trimethoprim-sulfamethoxazole, while combination therapy with antipseudomonal antibiotics (imipenem, meropenem, aztreonam) is used to ensure treatment of resistant strains. Of course, we should not neglect the possible side effects of antibiotics, especially to the gastrointestinal system (diarrhea). The diarrhea occurs due to eradication of the normal gut flora by the antibiotic and results in an overgrowth of infectious bacteria. Therefore, the patient has to follow a diet rich in lactobacillus, found in organic yogurt, or kefir. In case there is a lactose intolerance, lactobacillus is also available in pharmaceutical made capsules. Another side effect symptom involves inflammation of gingiva, giving an itching feeling in the oral cavity. Supplementation of B complex vitamins is quite helpful. Intramuscular abscess after it is surgically opened has to be cleaned up twice on a daily basis, as long as the patient follows an antibiotic medication. White blood cells (WBCs) count, erythrocyte sedimentation rate (ESR) and C-reactive protein (CRP) are laboratory evaluations that should be considered on a weekly basis. This follow up will provide details concerning the progress of inflammation. Fever is also a good sign of inflammatory response. Creatinokinase enzyme (CPK) is a biochemical marker that is also elevated, as a result of the repeated intramuscular injections; named as rhabdomyolysis effect. Lactate dehydrogenase (LDH) is another biochemical evaluation, raised in tissue inflammation and cellular damage. When the abscess heals, scar tissue will form, therefore, no more injections in that area.

Sometimes, when the abscess is localized into the gluteal area, the athlete is unable to perform a hip flexion. This particular movement happens during the negative-eccentric phase of the leg press for example, or the squat. The reason is because of the extensive intramuscular abscess that forces press against the sciatic nerve. The hip flexion stretches the sciatic nerve, giving a painful sensation. As well know from human anatomy, the particular nerve is the largest in the peripheral nervous system. When sciatic nerve undergoes irritation, pain reflects on the head of the fibula; the bone located on the outer area of tibia. As the sciatic nerve proceeds down to the posterior femoral region, it splits into the posterior tibial nerve and the peroneal nerve.

Rarely, poor septic conditions (needle sharing, reusing needles and syringes) are responsible for the entrance of microbes into the muscle. Pure ethanol 95% must be used for sterilization of epidermis, both before and after the shoots. Of course we have to change the needles and better to use another syringe, in case we shoot on different areas on the same day. Subcutaneous injections are rarely to develop any kind of infection, since the adipose tissue has lesser amount of vessels and contamination spreads slower. Peptides are usually injected into the fat, as somatropin (human growth hormone- hGH), insulin and human chorionic gonadotropin.

Personally, I have once experienced a localized inflammation, dealing with a subcutaneous injection of hGH. It was something inevitable, since I had not followed strictly the sterilization circumstances and wrongly used the same needle twice. According to my personal experience, as a former steroid abuser during my bodybuilding competitive career, I faced two intramuscular abscesses, that both had to be surgically opened, while I was following an effective combination of antibiotics. For the first time, I decided to switch from the pharmaceutical brand (Winstrol Depot-Desma) of stanozolol, manufactured in Spain. Instead, I wrongly chose to use an underground product of Biogen labs. After a couple of weeks, both my deltoid and gluteus were infected, giving a feeling of discomfort and nausea. At first, I tried to self-care at home, by applying the initial steps of abscess treatment; but there was no progress. I was lucky that it was during my residency practice at the hospital, so I was treated successfully by my colleagues. General surgeon's cooperation, along with biopathologists, helped me to heal within four weeks. I fondly remember during the surgical procedure, the smell of burning flesh, as doctors were trying to stop the excessive bleeding. As I was told later, the steroid abuse costed me in terms of blood coagulation, so my bleeding time was prolonged (INR>1.3). In such cases,

Bodybuilding

vitamin K and plasma factors are administrated IV. Two years later, during my final competition at the Masters Nationals, there was a visible scar on my buttocks, although I was pretty well tanned and colored by spray.

ERYTHROPOIESIS AND ATHLETIC PERFORMANCE

One way to increase the aerobic capacity-resistance of an athlete ($VO_{2,\ max}$), is to enhance erythropoiesis. Studies have shown that one gram of hemoglobin (Hb) can bind ~ 1.34 ml of 0_2.

Thus, an increased amount of Hb also increases the amount of O_2 that can be delivered to the tissues. Moreover, the O_2 transport capacity and maximal O_2 uptake ($VO_{2,\ max}$) in athletes directly correlate with aerobic performance. Therefore, the increase of hematocrit, hemoglobin and consequently myoglobin is a clear advantage for aerobic athletic performance. Myoglobin is a protein that binds oxygen and incorporates it into the skeletal-striated muscles. Moreover, this hemoprotein is capable of releasing O_2 during periods of hypoxia or anoxia.

The hematocrit can increases in the following ways:

1) by living at altitude of over 2000 meters for at least one month (four weeks). As known, in higher altitude the air is thinner and therefore the oxygen content is lower. This is a direct stimulus to the kidneys to produce the growth factor erythropoietin (EPO), which stimulates bone marrow and enhances erythropoiesis. Then the athlete with increased hemoglobin can train at sea level, where O_2 concentration is maximum.

2) by having a diet rich in beef-buffalo meat and supplementation by liver aminos, combined with intramuscular injections of cyanocobalamin, follate and liquid iron with ascorbate tablets. These ingredients (iron, vitamin B12, follate) are the main substrates that ensure hemoglobin's synthesis and enhance erythrocytosis.

3) by the use of androgens (testosterone and synthetic derivatives-AAS), that stimulate erythropoietin (EPO) release,

increase red bone marrow activity, iron incorporation into the red cells and consequently elevate hemoglobin-hematocrit.

4) by the use of synthetic erythropoietin (r-EPO), that enhances erythropoiesis process. The increased number of red blood cells transports more oxygen, thus raising oxygen levels in the tissues, particularly muscles.

Elevation of hematocrit above 54 % (hemoglobin>18) increases the risk for thrombotic stroke, pulmonary embolism or deep vein thrombosis. Therefore athletes should use salicylic acid (aspirin), which has a thrombolytic-antiplatelet action, against blood coagulation. The drug belongs to Non Steroid Anti-inflammatory Drugs (NSAIDs), that inhibit prostaglandins (PGs), through thromboxanes (TX) & cycloxygenase enzymes (COX1, COX2). Aspirin's action inactivates platelets' activity, not their absolute number.

Since the white fast-twitch fibers involved in explosive sports (bodybuilding, sprints, shot put, javelin, weightlifting) are rich in glycogen and poor in myoglobin, the use of r-EPO is meaningless. As a result, the increase of hematocrit and consequently hemoglobin-myoglobin, benefits the prolonged endurance events (marathon, cycling, triathlon).However, some elite sprinters (Tim Montgomery, Marion Jones) claimed that r-EPO gave them improved recovery within training sessions.

CORTICOSTEROIDS

Corticosteroids even though they are catabolic, they are included in the chemical enhancement of a professional cyclist or marathon runner, because of their anti-inflammatory activity and their ability to cure the musculoskeletal system, particularly the joints.

Additionally, corticosteroids and specifically glucocorticoids (cortisone) contribute to the release of immediate energy, through hyperglycemia, via gluconeogenesis in the liver.

Furthermore corticosteroids are first-line therapy for persistent asthma and severe chronic obstructive pulmonary disease (COPD) and anti-inflammatory medications for crisis prevention (reducing the frequency and severity of exacerbations).They improve respiratory function, reduce bronchial hyper responsiveness, control inflammation, increase the action of β 2-agonists, thus the maximum oxygen intake (by increasing Forced Expiratory Volume at 1 sec - FEV 1).

Cortisone is the major glucocorticosteroid, while aldosterone the basic mineral corticosteroid.The former is responsible of glycemia and the latter is involved in the regulation of electrolyte and water balance (sodium and water retention).

Long term use of corticosteroids can lead to insulin resistance, tendon rupture, osteopenia-osteoporosis, gastric ulcer, psychotic events, hypertension, susceptibility to microbial and fungal infections, adrenal insufficiency and secondary hypogonadism in men.Chronic administration may also lead to drug-induced (secondary) Cushing's syndrome with central obesity particularly of the trunk and face (JFK's moon face).

Cortisol blockers are drugs that inhibit the catabolic effect of cortisol. Aminoglutethimide is an anti-steroid drug that blocks the conversion of cholesterol to pregnenolone and consequently decreases synthesis of all hormonally active steroids. Orimeten/Cytadren is medically prescribed for the treatment of hormone sensitive metastatic breast cancer.

However, potentially the drug can prevent muscle wasting. Thus it is abused by bodybuilders and other steroid users to lower circulating levels of cortisol in the body and prevent muscle loss.

Aminoglutethimide suppresses Hypothalamic-Pituitary-Adrenal (HPA) axis, therefore ACTH is stimulated from anterior pituitary. In order to prevent HPA axis distortion, we can either use aminoglutethimide on/off every other day, or to provide simultaneously injectable hydroxycortisone. Aminoglutethimine careless abuse can lead to secondary Addison's disease and severe adrenal insufficiency.Cortisol's crush would lead to hypotension, hypoglycemia, fatigue, abdominal pain, nausea, vomiting headache, confusion, lethargy.

STEROID LETHARGY EFFECT

Quite often competitive bodybuilders keep asking me, why they feel so exhausted, during the cutting phase. The answer is multifaceted and not simple and I explain it below:

the muscle strain, resulting to rhabdomyolysis effect, is great.

The muscle fibers break and myoglobin is released into the blood, while the muscles get inflamed. The creatine kinase (CPK) enzyme is increased at five times the levels of the normal limits (> 1000).

the calories consumed are low – as well as the carbohydrates - something that does not leave us much room for energy. The protein is not an immediate source of energy, and neither are fats in a ketogenic diet.

the anti-inflammatory hormone cortisol is suppressed, since its concentration is inversely proportional to the AAS (especially the highly anabolic trenbolone), as with the b2 - stimulators (clenbuterol hydrochloride). Low cortisol along with overwork leads to supressed immune response, leading to a significant reduction of white blood cells (WBC's.). Therefore, the athlete often exhibits low grade fever and muscle aches.

estrogens are suppressed, linked to several different adverse effects.

- Moodiness (beta estradiol is linked to serotonin - the hormone of joy).

- Poor libido, since both sexes need both kinds of steroid hormones for good libido.

- Low levels of IGF1, since insulin that promotes the release of somatomedin C, is suppressed.

the intake of dietary cholesterol is low, thus the biosynthesis of endogenous testosterone and DHEA, remains low.

Therefore different parameters contribute to this clinical phenomenon, no matter that kind of supplements the athletes use.

When estrogens are low there is poor water retention (edema), leadind to inadequate muscle glycogen synthesis. This obviously costs in lesser strength and stamina for anaerobic physical activity (explosive resistance exercise).

As a solution I propose:

The increase of complex carbohydrates in the form of carb cycling, the increase of the anti-catabolic supplements (HMB, Bcaa's, glutamine), the increase of the MCT's as an alternative energy source, the abstain from any physical activity for 48 hours and massages to remove any accumulated lactic acid.But also the disscontinuation of the potent aromatase inhibitors for a couple of days, or their temporary replacement by SERM's and mesterolone to avoid aromatization.

Conclusively, a common occurrence that can be interpreted simplified as a result of hard dieting, has its deeper etiology in the principles of pathophysiology.

DIURETICS

Diuretics are a class of drugs increasing urine output by the kidney, thus prescribed against hypertension, left heart failure and pulmonary or systemic edema.

Furosemide is a powerful diuretic, available both in injectable and per os form. Furosemide is of immediate action and flushes urine within 20min.It works at the loop of Henle of kidney, inhibiting the sodium-potassium-chloride pump and leading to increased diuresis and natriuresis (increased sodium loss). The drug also induces renal synthesis of prostaglandins, which contributes to its renal action. Furosemide is capable of reducing all electrolytes and minerals, leading to hypokalemia, hyponatremia, hypocalcemia, hypomagnesemia, which is likely to cause cramps and metabolic alkalosis.

On the contrary, spironolactone is a potassium sparing diuretic. It belongs to the aldosterone inhibitors, a class of diuretics which antagonize the actions of aldosterone at the distal segment of the distal tubule.

Aldosterone is a hormone that belongs to the miniralcorticoids and is secreted by the adrenal cortex. It influences the reabsorption of sodium and excretion of potassium of the kidney, thus increasing water retention, blood pressure and blood volume. Because potassium is the principal intracellular ion, its retention (by spirolactone's action), will contribute to a better cellular volume, positively affecting the maintenance of the cellular size. Aldosterone plays an important role in the last week before a bodybuilding contest.

In order to inhibit aldosterone and eliminating water retention, we trick the body with an intentional increased intake of sodium chloride. This apparently will suppress any sodium retention the following days. Usually we quit from extra sodium intake, the very last day of glycogen depletion, just before the carb loading phase.

Abuse of spironolactone might lead to life threatening side effects, due to dramatic elevation of potassium (hyperkalemia) and metabolic acidosis. Myocardium is quite sensitive to this metabolic imbalance and can easily undergo severe arrhythmias (ventricular tachycardia, fibrillation) or even cardiac arrest.ECG changes in a patient with hyperkalemia are an ominous portent of potentially fatal arrhythmias.

The fact that the adrenal cortex produces a fair amount of dehydroepiandrosterone (DHEA), it is understandable, that abuse of spironolactone will lead to dose-dependent gynecomastia. The anti-androgenic property of spironolactone (breast tenderness and enlargement) is even more apparent in women who lack the gonads (testicles) and substantially their testosterone is produced by the ovaries and adrenals. Women use spironolactone in order to reduce the aesthetic androgenic side effects of androgenic anabolic steroids (AAS), specifically hirsutism. Spironolactone acts suspensively on the steroid hormone synthesis and leads to hypogonadism with decreased sperm count and motility. Spironolactone is not of immediate action and stable concentrations are achieved within almost three days of treatment initiation. For better metabolism, the dosage should be splitted into am/pm timing. The appropriate timing for spironolactone's use would be the very first day of carb depletion phase. Potassium rich foods (bananas or potatoes) are strictly prohibited. Spironolactone should get gradually reduced in order to avoid any possible rebound effect. The most efficient method in order to achieve the best results of diuretics should be the combination of potassium sparing and non potassium sparing diuretics, hence spironolactone and furosemide. However, dosages should be reduced to half.

Diuretics are extremely dangerous substances, responsible of hypovolemia and dehydration, spasms of striated muscles (cramps), hypotension (a drop of systemic blood pressure) and severe arrhythmias.

A notable example of the cardiovascular collapse caused by abuse of diuretics was the tragic death of "the giant killer", Arab Mohamed Benaziza (Momo) at the Dutch grand prix in 1993.Not only he abused spironolactone, but he also quitted from water intake and consumed clenbuterol in powder form, according to his close friend, Sammir Bannout.

Diuretics are preferably used before night sleep, in order to avoid any possible fainting episode, due to hypotension. Potatoes and bananas, rich in potassium, can help in case of hypokalemia.

Diuretics are useful in the days of carbohydrate overload to avoid the risk of possible water retention under the skin.The morning of the contest, in case there is still water retention, the combination of a moderate dose of furosemide (10mg) along with spironolactone (12.5mg), is a safe way to eliminate extra water. Note that dehydrated muscles are not capable of proper contraction.

In such cases, calcium tablets and liquid magnesium are good choices.

AROMATASE INHIBITORS

Aromatase inhibitors (AIs) are a class of drugs used in breast cancer. Inhibiting the action of the enzyme aromatase, which converts androgens into estrogens, AIs suppress estrogen production and are considered as potent anti estrogens. The inactivation of the aromatase enzyme found in high concentration in subcutaneous-adipose tissue, is the mechanism of their action.

AIs basically inhibit estrogen production, in contrast to the old generation of antiestrogens the Selective Estrogen Receptors Modulators (SERMs). SERMs occupy the estrogenic receptors, thus making the circulating estrogens unable to attach to the receptors.

The two types of AIs include suicidal steroidal inhibitors, such as exemestane and non-steroidal inhibitors, such as anastrozole and letrozole. Exemestane prevents the rise of estradiol (E2) for quite a while, after its being used. The drug almost suppresses plasma and tissue estrogen level (estradiol-E2) by 85% in vivo of total estrogen.

Aromatase inhibitors have several side effects, when abused on a daily basis (for aesthetic purposes).

1) AIs have a significant negative impact on atheromatic index thus increasing the risk of cardiovascular disease. Studies have shown an increase in total cholesterol (TC) and low-density lipoprotein (LDL) cholesterol levels and a decrease in high-density lipoprotein (HDL) cholesterol levels.

2) They lower bone mineral density (BMD), by lowering osteoblastic activity, resulting in increased risk of skeletal fragility.

Therefore, arthritis, osteoarthritis, arthralgias and osteopenia-osteoporosis are serious negative adverse events.

3) Estrogens and aromatisation lead to edema that lubricate synovial cavity in joints. Therefore, estrogens deprivation would cause joint stiffness and joint pain.

4) Estrogens are linked to the feeling of well being, due to their relation to serotonin, the hormone of joy. Therefore, AIs have a negative effect on mood.

5) Estrogens are necessary for sexual drive.

Lowering beta estradiol dramatically, would cost in libido.

6) Estrogens lead to water retention, known as edema.

Muscle glycogen synthesis is formed from starch and water.Consequently, without water retention, there is lack of muscle glycogen and pumping. This costs in terms of energy and muscle flexing.

7) Finally estrogens improve androgens receptors (AR) affinity.

This was demonstrated by scientists who castrated male rats. As a result of this, estrogens went sky high. Afterwards male rats were given methyltrienolone AAS (M3) and the bonding between the steroid molecule and the AR was 500 times stronger. In a study held by Greeks in Aretaion University Hospital, 1mg/day of anastrozole or 2.5 mg/day of letrozole for 6 months could elevate LH and TT, through lower beta estradiol (E2).Letrozole is even more potent than anastrozole, while exemestane is considered to be a suicidal AI. However, AIs abuse will crush on E2, which will have reverse effects in libido. A small amount of estrogens is required for proper sexual drive.Besides, AIs abuse will have a negative impact on high-density lipoprotein (HDL) and bone mineral density (BMD).Joints also tend to ache, due to less lubrication.

ARTHRALGIA OF AROMATASE INHIBITORS

Aromatase inhibitors (AIs) are an important component of the treatment of hormone receptor-positive breast cancer in females. At the same time, they are necessary to prevent aromatization (estrogenic activity) caused by androgenic anabolic steroids (AAS).

The first class of anti-estrogenic drugs are Selective Estrogen Receptors Modulators (SERM's), which act selectively in certain tissues (tamoxifen, clomiphene), occupying the estrogenic receptors, thus making circulating estrogens unable to attach to the receptors.

Modern aromatase inhibitors include suicidal steroidal inhibitors (exemestane) and non-steroidal inhibitors (anastrozole, letrozole), which inhibit the action of aromatase enzyme that converts androgens to estrogens. Aromatization takes place in a variety of tissues, such as mammary gland, adipose tissue, liver and brain.These drugs have the ability to diminish peripheral-circulating estrogens and beta estradiol (E2) in particular.E2 is the main representative of estrogens. During a precontest preparation, or "cutting phase" AIs are widely abused.

This leads to a plethora of different side effects, with "arthralgia of aromatase inhibitors" being a common toxicity. The symptoms include joint pain, with most frequent in the wrists, knees, ankles, elbows and shoulders. This discomfort is usually symmetrical. Other symptoms include morning stiffness, muscle pain, skull and neck aching, carpal tunnel syndrome and restricted mobility of the affected part. The average time of the appearance of symptoms is about 4 weeks.Studies showed significantly higher rates of carpal tunnel syndrome following the use of anastrozole and exemestane compared to tamoxifen. Laboratory tests and imaging examinations are normal and necessary to exclude conditions that require immediate attention, such as traumatic, inflammatory, autoimmune arthritis, fracture, mechanical derangement, or tumor.

The pathogenic mechanism of AIs -induced arthralgia has different origins:

Firstly, we know that estrogens and aromatisation particularly, are associated with water retention and edema.

This is a beneficial environment for the synovial cavity, since joints are lubricated, and thus friction is diminished.

Moreover, studies have shown that estrogens are natural pain inhibitory receptors, an evolutionary adaptation to help women to better tolerate the pain during childbirth, when estrogen levels are particularly high.

Thus estrogen deprivation makes the body more vulnerable to pain sensation and decreases threshold for painful stimuli. The perception of pain is more intense. Scientific evidence shows that, AIs do not cause actual harm to the joint destruction of articular surfaces, cartilage, ligaments and muscles surrounding. Therefore, discontinuation of the AIs leads to prompt relief of symptoms.

The most appropriate intervention for pain management in AIs-associated arthralgia may be a combination of pharmacologic approaches in conjunction with dietary supplements for bone protection.

As an alternative treatment the use of SERMs is proposed, since these drugs act selective estrogenic on the liver and anti-estrogenic on the breast tissue. Tamoxifen occupies the estradiol receptor, without blocking the action of aromatase enzyme in the breast and subcutaneous tissues.

Estrogens still can circulate in blood, therefore synovial cavity of joints do not become dry.

The use of hyaluronic acid in liquid form acts as a moisturizer, when combined with hydrolyzed collagen.

Also glucosamine-chondroitin-MSM complex helps. These are glycoproteins, which moisturize the articular surfaces and the hyaline cartilage. The use of ascorbic acid in ester form of vitamin C contributes to the biosynthesis of collagen protein.

Non-steroidal anti-inflammatory drugs (NSAIDs), on the one hand suppress the inflammation and pain, since they inhibit inflammatory cytokines (prostaglandins).On the contrary, they sabotage the phenomenon of muscle inflammation and also account for increased risk of upper gastrointestinal bleeding (stomach, duodenum).As an alternative, omega 3 PUFAs (DHA/EPA) coming from fish oil may be used.

AROMATASE INHIBITORS AND VISUAL DISORDERS

Estrogens directly affect a wide range of bodily functions, with positive and negative effects depending on the targeted organ. Estrogen receptors exist in various organs, including the anterior and posterior segment of the eye and lacrimal gland. Thus, changes in estrogenic activity affect the visual function both centrally (optic nerve) and distally.

Selective Estrogen Receptors Modulators (SERMs) such as tamoxifen and clomiphene act on the estrogen receptors and may exert agonistic or antagonistic activity, depending on the targeted tissue. In the eye, they have the ability to inhibit the action of estrogens, causing various symptoms.

These include flashing lights (photopsia), blurred vision, color perception changes (dyschromatopsia), increased sensitivity to light (photophobia),images in the visual field, reduced peripheral vision and scotomas.

A rare but serious complication is "tamoxifen retinopathy", a disturbancewhich depends on the total cumulative dose of the drug.It is characterized by bilateral presence of crystalline deposits in the retina with or without macular edema. Tamoxifen can also induce cataracts.

As known, aromatase inhibitors (AIs) are a class of drugs that inhibit the action of the enzyme aromatase, which converts androgens into estrogens. Thus, AIs suppress estrogen production and are considered potent anti estrogens in the peripheral tissues.The two types of AIs include suicidal steroidal inhibitors, such as exemestane and non-steroidal inhibitors, such as anastrozole and letrozole.

Ocular side effects occur rarely and are linked to retinal hemorrhage, retinal detachment and disorders in color vision, similar to those caused by SERM's. The side effects of SERMs and AI in the eye are dose and time dependent. It should be noted that, the ocular toxicities of tamoxifen such as macular edema or retinal deposits are often reversible, if the drug is discontinued or the dosage reduced.

But, as with all medicines, every individual's susceptibility plays also a role, just like the rest of the eye concurrent problems (dry eye, myopia-short sighted, increased intra-ocular pressure) do too. Therefore, the use of SERMs and AI should be stopped immediately after the occurrence of visual disturbances and a full ophthalmologic monitoring should follow.

ESTROGEN FACTS

The presence of estrogens is beneficial for the atherosclerotic profile. This is the reason why women have lower mortality in heart attacks. Therefore, the lower estrogens one has, the worse the ratio of HDL/LDL is.

On the other hand, too much of estrogens, are linked to increased thrombosis and furthermore estrogens are a negative feedback for Hypothalamic Pituitary Testicular Axis (HPTA) and GnRH. It is well known that women, who use contraceptive pills, have a higher risk for thrombotic episodes and should use salicylic acid, or fish oil.

The more aromatized an anabolic is, the higher its anabolic character is. Oxymetholone and methandrostenolone are two examples of 17 alkalized anabolic pills with a high estrogenic capacity. Other AAS, used during bulking (off season) are boldenone (Equipose) and nandrolone (Decadurabolin). Both of them have a moderate estrogenic activity.

Estrogens have a significant role in muscle development. Estrogens make androgen receptors more receptive to the anabolic molecule. This was shown in a study, where scientists castrated male guinea pigs and then granted them the powerful anabolic steroid 17 alkylated pill, methyltrienolone (M3). With their castration, the mice dramatically increased estrogens' levels and eliminated their androgens. It was observed that the link between M3 and receptors was 500% more powerful than before their castration. Insulin like growth factor (IGF1) is a peptide responsible for muscle development and regeneration of the cartilage.

It is known, that among the factors for GH release, is the presence of E2. The concentration of somatomedin C decreases as estrogens are reduced.

Aromatisation is a process that promotes the presence of the IGF1 peptide.

Therefore, the fewer estrogens we have, the less production of the anabolic hormone will be. The use of tamoxifen citrate (SERM) has a negative impact on IGF1 production in the liver.

Proof that estrogens are an anabolic agent and contribute to weight gain and muscularity through water retention and glycogen, is the fact that one of the strongest 17 alkalized AAS, fluoxymesterone, with an anabolic ratio 18 times greater than testosterone and 9 times more anabolic than oxymetholone, yet is not used for weight gain itself, but to increase muscle strength, hardness and density.

GYNECOMASTIA

By the term gynecomastia, we mean the accumulation of adipose tissue beneath the mammary gland, leading to breast tenderness and enlargement in the male. This term is often used by bodybuilders, due to accumulated estrogens under the nipple (areola).

Estrogen levels that are in imbalance with testosterone levels (increased ratio of of estrogens/androgens) are responsible for the development of gynecomastia.furthermore, estrogens can increase serum levels of sex hormone binding globulin (SHBG), which binds free testosterone (the active form-FT), leading to decreased levels of FT and testosterone's action in male mammary gland.

Medications which can cause gynecomastia include:

- Androgenic-anabolic steroids (AAS) converted to estrogens (beta estradiol) by the enzyme aromatase. Estrogenic AAS are: Oxymetholone depending on aromatization environment, Nandrolone, Equipose, Testosterone, Methandienone and Methyltestosterone.

- Finasteride, an anti-androgen used in the treatment of benign prostate hyperplasia (BPH).

- Spironolactone, a diuretic with anti-androgenic property, can produce dose-dependent gynecomastia.

The fact that the adrenal cortex produces a fair amount of dehydroepiandrosterone (DHEA), it is understandable, that abuse of spironolactone will lead to gynecomastia.

- Ranitidine/Cimetidine: used in the treatment of duodenal ulcer

- Opioids pain killers: codeine

Bodybuilding

- Marijuana (weed, pot)

- Barbiturates: Diazepam (valium)

Initially, the problem is addressed by reducing weight and lowering body fat percentage, accompanied by resistance training. If there is no improvement, the athlete should undergo a hormonal blood panel (beta estradiol, estriol, estrone and prolactine), which could reveal any supraphysiological serum levels of these hormones. Accordingly, he should use an anti-estrogen (tamoxifen with mesterolone, or aromatase inhibitors, such as anastrozole, letrozole and exemestane). Dopamine agonists sich as cabergoline and bromocriptine, will lower porlactinemia. If the problem persists, then the gland should be removed surgically (mastectomy). Liposuction is a surgical procedure, which removes breast fat, but not the breast gland tissue itself.

SELECTIVE ANDROGEN RECEPTOR MODULATORS

Selective Androgen Receptor Modulators (SARMs) are a new class of anabolic agents. They are considered are supplements with anabolicproperties, banned from WADA/USADA and IOC.Their chemical structure is not of a steroidal molecule,as with AAS.

As their name implies, they have selective role in androgenic receptors. Meaning they don't harm certain tissues with androgenic receptors, such as prostate,scalp,skin.

However, they are supposed to bind the androgens receptor and have potent anabolic effect.Therefore, they act as strong anabolics with minimal androgenic side effects.Among them,ostarine is the most popular (MK 2866).Other SARMs include Andrarine,Ligandrol,Enobiosarm,RAD140 and the YK 11.

From my personal experience,that involves reports of my patients,the conclusion was that these substances are not as innocent and harmless, as some speculate.There are specific deviations in laboratory results, showing that SARMs are hepatotoxic,HPTAsuppressive and atherogenic.

Transaminemia (AST,ALT >100) reveals their hepatotoxicity.LH, TT, FTsuppression shows that they lower endogenous testosterone production.

While HDL drops means they can lead in the long term to cardiovascular disease.

In reality, there are quite familiar findings with 17 alkylated orals. ThereforeI am quite skeptical and suspicious, regarding how legit they are.

Bodybuilding

Moreover, Andrarine is reported to cause visual disturbances, such as blurred vision. Probably due to retina's disturbances, or cornea's.

Considering these facts, SARMs are suggested not to be used more than a two months period, while tapering of their dosage ensures the HPTA suppressive effects are minimal.

MEDICAL INDICATIONS FOR THERAPEUTIC ADMINISTRATION OF PEDs

Indications for therapeutic administration of androgenic anabolic steroids (AAS) are: hypogonadism, osteopenia-fractures, muscle wasting-cachexia syndrome associated with HIV infection (AIDS), breast cancer, burn injury, severe aplastic anemia and other myelodysplastic syndromes, the congenital angioedema and sarcopenia in the elderly.

AAS have beneficial effects on bone mineral density, through direct interaction with osteoblasts and by enhancing calcium reabsorption in renal tubules leading to calcium retention. There are also reports of positive effects on fracture healing, on lubrication of synovial cavities, as well as on nitrogen balance in polytrauma patients. Some AAS can increase erythropoietin (EPO) production from the kidneys, iron absorption and also stimulate the production of red cells from bone marrow, improving erythropoiesis process.

Other AAS are used to reverse wasting complications associated with HIVinfection (> stage 1-WHO classification) and cancer, by improving protein synthesis and restoration of lean body mass. During tumors specific proteins known as cachexins are responsible of symptoms of cachexia and muscle catabolism.

It is important to note that, testosterone replacement therapy has beneficial effect in mood and cognitive function in hypogonadal men and patients with Alzheimer's disease.

In medicine, performance enhancing drugs are used for therapeutic purposes in the following conditions:

- Anastrozole, letrozole, exemestane (aromatase inhibitors): breast cancer

Bodybuilding

- Tamoxifen citrate (SERM): breast cancer

- Clomiphen citrate (SERM): promotion of ovarian rupture and ovulation phase

- Fluoxymesterone (androgen): advanced breast cancer, osteoporosis

- Oxymetholone (anabolic): severe aplastic anemia, wasting complications associated with HIV

- Stanozolol (anabolic): angioedema, muscular dystrophy

- Methandrostenolone (anabolic): post traumatic syndrome

- Oxandrolone (anabolic): delayed puberty, AIDScachexia

- Methenolone enanthate (anabolic): muscle weakness and wasting

- Nandrolone undecaonate (anabolic): osteoporosis and complications (fractures)

- Drostanolone propionate (anabolic-androgenic): advanced inoperable breast cancer

- Testosterone enanthate/cypionate/undecaonate/propionate (androgen): hypogonadism (primary, secondary, late onset hypogonadism), Kleinefelter syndrome, muscular dystrophy

- Mesterolone (androgen): erectile dysfunction, depression

- Ephedrine HCL (vasoconstrictor): allergic rhinitis

- Clenbuterol HCL (b-2 agonist, bronchodilator): asthma, chronic obstructive pulmonary disease

-Somatropin-HGH (growth hormone): growth hormone deficiency (primary and secondary), short stature at birth with no catch-up growth, AIDS induced cachexia

- Insulin: insulin dependent diabetes mellitus I (DM 1)

- Human chorionic gonadotropin (HCG): cryptorchidism in puberty, IVF procedures

- Fourosemide (diuretic): chronic heart failure, hypertension

- Erythropoietin (EPO): anemia in chronic renal failure (dialysis), neoplasms

- Thyroxine/T4, triiodothyronine/T3 (thyroid hormones): Hypothyroidism, Hashimoto thyroiditis

- Aminoglutethimide (adrenal steroid-cortisol inhibitor): Cushing's syndrome, hormone sensitive metastatic breast cancer

- Metformin: diabetes mellitus II (DM 2), polycystic ovary syndrome

POST CYCLE THERAPY (PCT)

After the end of an anabolic androgenic steroid (AAS) cycle, the steroid user should estimate the half life of the particular esters he used.This will define the correct timing of drug clearance in the system. Depending on the slow or fast esters, one or two weeks approximately are required in order to eliminate the substance from the body. The idea of the gradual reduction of injectable testosterone does not provide any benefit to the hormonal system. It only reinforces the belief that the user is still on a cycle. Either one reduces the dose gradually or abruptly-cold turkey, the Hypothalamic Pituitary Testicular Axis (HPTA) is shut off from day one (when testosterone is used).

The first phase of PCT involves the administration of beta-human chorionic gonadotropin (beta-HCG)peptide that will ensure stimulation of HPTA. HCG is produced from the placenta after implantation, during the early stages of pregnancy.

Actually prediction test of pregnancy is checked out by serum, or urine levels of HCG.It is a mimicker-analogue of luteinizing hormone (LHRH) that stimulates endogenous testosterone production in the Leydig cells of the testicles. It is obvious that HCG, as a gonadotropin, will inhibit GnRH in the hypothalamus.It helps during primary hypogonadism, when hypophysis is active (LH/FSH normal or high levels), while Total (TT) and Free Testosterone (FT) are low.

All AAS suppress the HPTA. Therefore, the endogenous testosterone production is reduced significantly (homeostatic mechanism).

The use of HCG permits testicles and scrotum to keep their volume and triggers endogenous testosterone production. The usual protocol provides the intramuscular-subcutaneous injections of 1500 IU every third day (72 hours) for two, or three weeks. Usually the dosage of 5000 IU is used for cases of cryptorchidism in boys who have not yet entered puberty and in IVF procedures.

Initially all AAS users suffer from primary hypogonadism, which gradually turns into secondary (late onset). Abuse of beta hCG(> 5000 IU) and its extensive use (over four weeks) will cause testicle whipping and saturation of LH receptors. The resulting rise in natural testosterone will inhibit its own production on the hypothalamus and pituitary gland and eventually will have a negative impact.

The prolonged HCG abuse for over four weeks could lead to high levels of estradiol with peripheral edema, gynecomastia, and weight gain, mood swings with emotional instability and headaches due to increased intracranial pressure from water retention.

We should concern that a peptide from chemical point of view, does not aromatise.However, as LH will increase endogenous testosterone production, this testosterone will eventually get aromatised.

The second phase of PCT involves clomiphene citrate, a medication belonging to the class of Selective Estrogen Receptors Modulators (SERMs).This compound acts half estrogenic and the other half as anti-estrogenic. Clomiphene is attached to their receptor. Clomiphene's actual action is to trick hypothalamus, by giving the sensation of decreased estrogens. The drop in estrogens would signal for GnRH release from hypothalamus, thus stimulating LH & FSH production fromhypophysis. Therefore, we realise that this mechanism is opposite than how beta-HCG works.

Along with clomiphene citrate, another SERM (tamoxifen citrate) can also be used simultaneously. It lowers beta estradiol (E2) in the blood and this is a positive signal for GnRH and LH, FSH production. SERMs are also used for two to three weeks long. Tapering is the usual dosage (50mg=>25mg & 20mg=>10mg). The fact that clomiphene acts estrogenically to other tissues (brain) explains the fact that the medication may cause dysthymia (moodiness). In the liver, aromatisation by SERMs improves atheromatic profile and ratio of lipoproteins HDL/LDL. Occasionally, after the discontinuation of SERMs, estrogens might rise.

HORMONAL REPLACEMENT THERAPY (HRT) AS A RESULT OF ANDROGEN INDUCED HYPOGONADISM (AIH-AAS ABUSE)

As we age, our hormonal profile corresponds to the process of ageing. In both sexes, steroid hormones, androgens and estrogens are reduced and the typical midlife crisis exists, menopause and andropause.

After the age of 35, the average age-related reduction in total testosterone is 10% per decade. The symptoms that characterize andropause syndrome are: depression-melancholy, decline in cognitive function (foggy mind), decreased libido and energy, erectile dysfunction, decreased Bone Mineral Density (BMD) - osteopenia, reduced muscle mass and strength-sarcopenia, fatigue, weakness, gynecomastia and increased visceral-omental abdominal fat.

Does andropause lead to depression? Absolutely yes. Absence of androgens and DHT002Clead to low self esteem and poor sex drive. On the other hand,testosterone will optimize neurotransmitter like serotonin (the joy hormone) and dopamine (feeling of reaward).Physicians widely prescribe medications in order to treat depression (SSRIs),that lead to prolactinemia and anorgasmia.So the problem is not solved from its origin.Similarly urologist widely prescribe 5PDEi in order to treat erectile dysfunction,however the lack of libido still remains. Again the problem isn't approached from where it initiates. In the bottom line society doesn't want testosterone. Obviously because it of low expence and can help against a variety of diseases. Consider that menopause and HRT were widely spread in women since the late 80s,while gynecologists and internal medicine pathologists were in charge of it. On the contrary andropause is still considered as a taboo subjet,because it affects mans pride and ego;having to do with his erectile dysfunction. In Europe we used to have the so called hormonophobia,meaning the fear of hormones,based on ignorance. Hopefully this has changed the past decade,now that we are aware and the wave of TRT/HRT in men spreads rapidly worldwide. Antiageing and age management strategies have not being part of the classic academic lesson in medical schools. Enhaging fileds of pathology,,urology and endocrinology.The most important thing is not just to follow the book,but to walk your theory;otherwise you are missing half of the truth based on hard earned experience. In this way you're more than a regular MD and more of another bro scientist who preaches online.

The majority (98%) of testosterone is bound to Sex Hormone Binding Globulin (SHBG), a protein that transportstestosterone into the blood serum. A very small percentage (2%) remains free in unbound form. The higher rate of free-bioavailable testosterone (FT) is free, the higher the libido and muscle strength will be. Therefore, free testosterone and SHBG values are inversely proportional. Only free testosterone binds to the androgen receptor (AR) in the cytoplasm.

As we age, serum levels of SHBG increase and free testosterone decrease, which represent one of the laboratory findings of andropause. This is justified by the sarcopenia-cachexia-muscle wasting and concurrently the increase of the subcutaneous fat and adipose tissue that elevates serum levels of beta estradiol (E2) .Therefore, the elevation of beta-estradiol (E2) increases SHBG and reduces the FT.

Hormone replacement therapy (HRT) is one of the parameters of proper age management, thus contributing to the hormonal balance of the middle-aged crisis. Each subject with hypogonadism should be individually studied and counseled after the evaluation of certain hormonal serum levels. Each case is unique and one size does not fit all.

Hormonal assessment includes levels of Lutelizing Hormone (LH), Follicle Stimulating Hormone (FSH), Total Testosterone (TT), Free Testosterone (FT), Sulfate Dihydroepiandrosterone (S-DHEA), Sex Hormone Binding Globulin (SHBG), Estradiol (E2) and Prolactine (PRL).

Primary hypogonadism is characterised by normal or elevated levels of LH, FSH, while total and free testosterone levels are low. This practically is translated into smaller testicles with normal spermatogenesis. In primary hypogonadism, we usually administrate HCG, followed by clomiphene citrate and tamoxifen citrate (SERMs) for a couple of weeks, in order to restore hypothalamic-pituitary-gonadal axis (HPTA).

Secondary hypogonadism is characterised by low levels of total and free testosterone associated with low levels of FSH and LH, since the patient's HPTA is shut off. S-DHEA is usually low.

"Late onset" hypogonadism (LOH) is a mixed (primary/secondary) form of hypogonadism, with a central (deficient GnRH and gonadotropin activity) and a peripheral (impaired steroidogenesis) component often simultaneously present.

Regarding androgenic-anabolic steroid (AAS) abusers, they initially develop primary hypogonadism, which gradually turns into secondary or late onset hypogonadism. This condition is also defined as "androgen induced hypogonadism", since it develops as a result of chronic abuse of AAS.

HPTA is a homeostatic mechanism, providing balance. Theadministration of exogenous steroid hormones will suppress HPTA's function, hence the endogenous hormone production. Time and dose of AAS abuse will result in testicular shrinkage eventually; this is a typical homeostatic mechanism, regulated from HPTA. Testosterone Replacement Therapy (TRT) is the solution to this hormonal defect. Considering that andropause exists after the age of fourty, HPTA is hardly to get restored with a regular Post Cycle Therapy protocol (HCG/SERMs). As a result, we should provide the appropriate amount of androgen, in order serum testosterone levels to be within the optimal range.

Before starting patients on HRT, doctors must rule out contraindications to treatment.Inhibitory, high-risk factors for potential adverse outcomes from hormone replacement therapy are:

- erythrocytosis (hemoglobin> 18)
- obstructive sleep apnea (OSA)
- benign prostatic hypertrophy (BPH=PSA> 4). The presence of a clinical prostatic carcinoma is contradictive to start HRT and should be carefully excluded by:

a. serum PSA/free PSA

b. pelvis MRI

c. digital rectal examination and

d. biopsy before starting any therapy.

- dyslipidemia with HDL <40

Testosterone could be administrated either intramuscularly (IM) or subcutaneous (SC) (parenterally), by gel- skin patch (transdermal), orally (per os), or even as a mucoadhesive buccal tablet. The testosterone esters that are used are usually of slow release , with enanthate and cypionate (70% release), while the decaonate is implemented with a larger dosage of 1000mg, having a slower half life release (60%).The frequency of intramuscular (IM) or subcutaneous (SC) injections varies from daily, twice weekly, weekly, or even every three months (testosterone undecaonate).Subcutaneous administration delays absorption and offers prolonged pharmacokinetics, due to lesser vascularity of fatty tissue. The suspicion that the administration of testosterone subcutaneously, would increase the chances of aromatization would valid for patients with a subcutaneous rate >15%.However, according to Dr.Justin Saya, the fact that testosterone is released from the ester after entering the bloodstream, breaks this claim. Therefore, increasing of beta estradiol (E2) does not occur by SC injections. The use of transdermal testosterone has beneficial effects on libido, since the skin has an increased concentration of the enzyme 5a reductase enzyme receptors.

In order to ensure proper spermatogenesis and testicular size, Human Chorionic Gonadotropin (hCG) is prescribed along with testosterone. As Dr. John Crisler mentions, a frequent small amount of HCG will mimic the natural testosterone production by Leydig cells in the testicles. According to Dr.Saya, hCG should be better used on the day before weekly administration. The day before the injection, serum testosterone levels will be lower. Therefore, the administration of hCG would give a boost and increase endogenous testosterone's production. According to papers of Nelson Vergel, author of the book "Testosterone, a man's guide", HCG use can provide a better hormonal environment for basic steroid hormones: pregnenolone, progesterone and dihydroepiandrosterone.

DHEA is a pro hormone, released by the adrenal glands, also called as "the mother of all hormones". In men, it is converted to estrone (E1), through androstenedione.Therefore in males, DHEA is slightly aromatised, especially in doses over 50mg per day. However DHEA, improves cognitive function, mood, libido, bone mineral density (BMD), body composition and provides prevention against cancer.

Testosterone is converted to estradiol, by the aromatase enzyme in adipose tissue, mammary gland, liver and brain. Therefore, anti-estrogens will ensure beta estradiol does not elevate above optimal range. E2 is necessary for proper libido, joints lubrication, muscle glycogen formation, proper BMD, well being feeling and Androgen Receptors affinity. However, estrogens should be within a certain range, as Dr.Crisler names it as "sweet spot".

Antiestrogens are usually Aromatase Inhibitors (AIs) such as anastrozole, letrozole, exemestane, or even the old generation of antiestrogens the Selective Estrogen Receptors Modulators (SERMs), such as tamoxifen citrate. Each individual has a different Estrogen Receptor (ER) affinity, therefore AIs dosage and frequency of use is strictly personalized.

It should be noted that, elevated levels of estrogen increase the risk of coagulopathy. Anti androgens, drugs that block the 5a reductase enzyme action, are better not to be used within HRT. Finasteride and dutasteride are responsible for dihydrotestosterone's (DHT) crush. Relative to testosterone, DHT is considerably more potent (5x times more in vivo). As known, testosterone is reduced to DHT by the enzyme 5a reductase.

One way to increase serum level value of free testosterone (FT), is the use of synthetic forms of DHT (mesterolone, drostanolone), or even danazol. Androgens bind tightly to SHBG, therefore more FT is able to circulate. DHT has beneficial effects on libido, self esteem, aggression, strength and cognitive function. However DHT is responsible for Benign Prostatic Hyperplasia (BPH) and Male Pattern Baldness (MPB) - androgenic alopecia. DHT receptors are located in scalp, epidermis and prostate gland. If someone has androgenic alopecia issues, or prostate hypertrophy, using 5a reductase inhibitors will improve both hair thinning and prostatic enlargement. However, the post finasteride syndrome (Post-Finasteride Syndrome by Dr John Crisler) is characterised by persistent sexual, neurological, and physical adverse reactions, such as depression, gynecomastia, chronic fatigue, increased fat deposition, obesity, erectile dysfunction and loss of sexual drive. In other words, a male feels like being castrated. According to the doctor, progesterone's use is beneficial and DHEA use might help.

The risks of testosterone replacement therapy depend upon age, life circumstances, and other medical conditions. These include:

- erythrocytosis (Hg>18 and Htc> 54%). Androgens stimulate erythropoiesis directly in the bone marrow, by promoting erythropoietin (EPO) synthesis in the kidney and by enhancing intestinal iron absorption from small intestine (jejunum-ileum), iron incorporation in red blood cells and hemoglobin synthesis.Erythrocytosis increases blood viscosity and the risk for thrombosis in the coronary, cerebrovascular, or peripheral circulation.This is the main reason for a frequent (every other day-twice per week) protocol, in order to avoid DHT & E2 spiking. Salicylic acid (aspirin) at 80mg is a preventive method against coagulation. For those who have G6PD enzymatic deficiency, the use of fish oil (DHA/EPA), will act on a similar way, as anti-thrombotic agent.

- the increased amount of testosterone (>150mg) leads to decreased levels of High Density Lipoprotein (HDL), which acts cardioprotective in arterial endothelium.

- worsening symptoms of benign prostatic hypertrophy.

Prostate cancer is not testosterone dependent after all.

According to late studies, what has been found in middle-aged people with prostatic cancer is a predominance of estrogen versus androgen, such as in obesity, or Metabolic Syndrome. Prostate cancer might be a contraindication in order to start hormone replacement, as a marginally increased level of prostate PSA antigen (BPH).

- worsening symptoms of sleep apnea, perhaps due to pharynx thickening .

Follow up assessment should be done four weeks (one month) after the beginning of TRT, in order to evaluate serum levels, until the patient reaches a stable hormonal environment. These include PSA/free PSA, hemoglobin, hematocrit, lipid profiles and should be also checked at three, six months and then annually. A digital rectal examination is necessary for those who are over fifty. Even better pelvicMRI that will reveal a 3D structure of the gland.

Also a BMD of lumbar spine or femoral neck should be measured every one to two years in hypogonadal men with osteoporosis, or low trauma fracture.

As Dr. John Crisler mentions: "the ultimate goal of TRT is to optimize health and happiness in patients, which means producing an environment where we have elevated testosterone to sufficient levels, with the body responding as if it is unaware of the exogenous manipulations".

SUPPRESSION OF THE PITUITARY-HYPOTHALAMIC-TESTICULAR AXIS, AS A RESULT OF AAS ABUSE

There is a homeostatic mechanism between hypothalamus-pituitary-testicles the Hypothalamic Pituitary Testicular Axis (HPTA), which is regulated interactively. Hypothalamus interacts with hypophysis, the pituitary gland located at the sella turcica of the sphenoid bone and gonads (testicles), adjusting their operation.

Androgenic anabolic steroids (AAS) are synthetic derivatives of testosterone, the main androgen. Testosterone itself significantly suppresses the HPTA axis, while several other derivatives induce the suppression into a greater or lesser extent.

In men, there is a homeostatic mechanism that interacts *AAS are classified into three main categories:*

Derivatives of testosterone (boldenone, fluoxymesterone, methyltestosterone)

Derivates of dihydrotestosterone-DHT (stanozolol, methenolone, oxandrolone, oxymetholone) and its synthetic forms (mesterolone, drostanolone)

Derivatives of the 19-nortestosterone (nandrolone, trenbolone)

Factors that contribute to the suppression of the HPTA axis are:

The origin of the AAS

Their degree of aromatization, namely their ability to produce estrogen (E2), through the aromatase enzyme in certain tissues (adipose tissue, mammary gland)

The duration and dosage of AAS abuse

The androgenicity of the particular AAS

AAS that cause the greatest suppression of the HPTA axis are:

Testosterone derivatives.

Testosterone itself, suppresses the axis from the very first day of use.

Highly aromatized AAS.

E2-beta estradiol provides a negative feedback to hypothalamus for GnRH production thatin turn will increase the production of LH (and testosterone) from the Leydig cells of testicles. Therefore, the AAS that aromatize or have a high affinity for the ER, (oxymetholone?, methyltestosterone, nandrolone, testosterone, methandienone), will suppress HPTA axis. Another reason why estrogens decrease the libido is the fact that, they increase the concentration of the sex hormone binding globulin (SHBG), which binds testosterone and leaves a small percentage to be released free as active form (FT).

Progestins (Nandrolone and its derivative trenbolone).

The derivatives of 19-nortestosterone have high progestational activity. This mainly occurs, under the presence of aromatisation and high beta estradiol concentration.Prolactin is a hormone released by frontal-anterior pituitary lobe, or adenohypophysis. It is inversely proportional to the production of testosterone. Therefore, prolactinemia will lead to suppression of the HPTA axis.

Potent androgens (fluoxymesterone, trenbolone, methyltrienolone).These drugs have a strong binding affinity to the androgen receptor (AR) in the brain.AAS cross the blood-brain barrier and bind tightly to the AR in hypothalamus (master gland in midbrain). This results in a greater suppression of the HPTA axis.

The androgenic activity-androgenicity of AAS is responsible for the development of the primary and secondary sexual characteristics (growth of testicles, scrotum, penis, prostate, pubic hair, voice deepening-hoarseness and the development of sebaceous glands).

Other biological actions of androgens include:

- Enhancement of erythropoiesis (by promoting erythropoietin synthesis in the kidney and by increasing erythroid colony-forming units in the bone marrow and promoting their differentiation into erythropoietin-responsive cells).

- Anabolic effect, i.e the increase of muscle mass and strength, increasing the size of muscle fibers. The administration of testosterone leads to

a) stimulation of aldosterone (mineral cocrticosteroid from adrenal cortex), responsible for sodium/natrium (and water retention)

b) positive nitrogen balance and

c) increased protein and contractile muscle tissue synthesis.

- Lipolysis (beta-oxidation of adipose tissue) by reducing abdominal fat, leading to lower the insulin resistance-increased sensitivity.

According to Dr.Michael Scally, author of book: "A question of muscle", AAS (that do not aromatise) could become the solution against obesity.

- Impact on the CNS with neurodegenerative effect, induction of apoptosis in hippocampus and enlargement of the amygdala.

Amydgala along with hippocampus belong to the limbic system, which

determines the emotional status. Clinical symptoms of AAS neurotoxicity include aggression, hypomania-mania, depression, bipolar disorder, psychotic behavior (misconceptions, delusions, and hallucinations)

AAS with high androgenicity, usually have high activity of 5a reductase enzyme and the produced DHT will mainly affect the prostate (hypertrophy-BPH) and scalp (alopecia-MPB). The DHT derivatives do not aromatize, thus don't lead to any water retention, or edema. Therefore, no beta estradiol (E2) is elevated, being responsible for the suppression of the HPTA axis (GnRH negative feedback). DHT is a potent androgen in the body (five times stronger than testosterone in vivo) and also suppressive to HPTA axis. At the same time, it is also anti-estrogenic, when applied topically (locally applied to male nipples having gynecomastia).Another fact demonstrating the antiestrogenic effect of DHT is when the use of 5a-reductase inhibitors (finasteride, dutasteride) for the treatment of prostatic hypertrophy or male pattern baldness. Men, who use this medication, later observe gynecomastia, depression and lack of libido (chemical castration). DHT is a strong androgen after all, and not a villain.

INDICATIVE AAS CYCLES

INDICATIVE CYCLE FOR BULKING

Week 1-4:

Testosterone blend (Sustanon-Ominadren): 2x weekly

Nandrolone decaonate (Decadurabolin):2x weekly

Oxymetholone (Anadrol 50):50 mg x2 am/pm, with breakfast and before training sublingually daily use

HGH 4IU subcutaneously first thing in the morning & 4IU post workout

5 IU fast-acting insulin after breakfast &5 IU postworkout (about 30 min opened window from usingHGH). In case IGF1 is used (insulin-like growth factor), 50mcg after training (instead of insulin).

Thyroxine (T4) 25mcg, 20min before breakfast

Mesterolone (Proviron):25 mg x2 am/pm, with breakfast and preworkout

Anastrozole (Arimidex):1 mg 3x weekly

Cabergoline (Dostinex): 0,5 mg 2x weekly

Metformin (Glucophage):500mg daily

Bodybuilding

Week 5-8:

Testosterone enanthate (Testoviron):2x weekly

Equipose (Ganabol-boldenone undecyclanate): 2x weekly

Methandienone (Dianabol):10 mg x4 am/pm, with breakfast, lunch, preworkout and dinner sublingually every day

HGH 4IU first thing in the morning & 4IU post workout

5IU fast acting insulin after breakfast & 5IU postworkout (30 minutes window, post to the HGH use)

Thyroxine (T4) 25mcg, 20min before breakfast

Mesterolone (Proviron): 25 mgx2 am/pm, with breakfast and preworkout

Anastrozole (Arimidex): 1 mg 3x weekly

Week 9-12:

Testosterone cypionate: 2x weekly

Trenbolone enanthate: 2x weekly

Fluoxymesterone (Halotestin): 10 mgx2 am/pm, with breakfast and preworkout sublingually used

HGH 4IU first thing in the morning & 4IU post workout

5IU fast acting insulin after breakfast & 5IU post workout (30 minutes window afterthe HGH use).

In case there is available insulin-like growth factor,50mcg right after training (instead of insulin)

Thyroxine (T4) 25mcg,20min before breakfast

Mesterolone (Proviron):25 mg x2 am/pm,with breakfast and before training)

Anastrozole (Arimidex): 1mg x3 weekly

Cabergoline (Dostinex): 0.5 mgx2 weekly

-Dosages are purely subjective!

-The treatment is <u>not</u> intended for therapeutic purposes.

-PCT with beta hCG, clomiphene, tamoxifen

Bodybuilding

INDICATIVE CYCLE FOR CUTTING

Week 1-4:

Testosterone blend (Sustanon-Omnadren): 2x weekly
Methenolone enanthate (Primobolan depot): 2x weekly
Parabolan: 2x weekly
HGH 4IU first thing in the morning, 30min before breakfast
500mg of metformin (Glucophage) with breakfast
Thyroxine (T4) 25mcg, 20min before breakfast
25mg ephedrine HCL-200mg of caffeine-300mg aspirin before training (ECA stack)
20mcg clenbuterol HCL with breakfast and 20mcg with lunch
Anastrozole (Arimidex): 1mg every day
Mesterolone (Proviron): 25 mg am/pm, with breakfast and before training

Week 5-8:

Testosterone propionate (Virormone): 3x weekly
Drostanolone propionate (Masteron): 3x weekly
Trenbolone acetate: 4 x weekly
HGH 4IU first thing in the morning, 30min before breakfast
500mg metformin (Glucophage) with breakfast
Thyroxine (T4) 25mcg, 20min before breakfast

25mg ephedrine HCL-200mg of caffeine-300mg aspirin before training (ECA stack)

20mcg clenbuterol HCL with breakfast &20mcg with lunch

Letrozole (Femara): 2,5 mg every day

Mesterolone (Proviron): 25 mg am/pm, with breakfast & before training

Week 9-10

Testosterone suspension(Aquaviron water based) preworkout

Drostanolone propionate (Masteron): x3 times weekly

Trenbolone suspension (base) preworkout

Stanozolol injection (Winstrol depot) preworkout

HGH 4IU first thing in the morning,30min before breakfast

500mg metformin (Glucophage) with breakfast

Thyroxine (T4) 25mcg, 20min before breakfast

25mg ephedrine HCL-200mg of caffeine-300mg aspirin before training (ECA stack)

20mcg clenbuterol HCL & 20mcg with lunch

Mesterolone (Proviron): 25 mg am/pm, with breakfast &before training.

Bodybuilding

Week 11-12:

Fluoxymesterone (Halotestin): 10 mgx4 am/pm with breakfast, lunch, before training, dinner sublingually used

Stanozolol per os (Winstrol tabs 2mg): 10 mgx4 am/pm with breakfast, lunch, before training, dinner sublingually used

Oxandrolone (Anavar tabs 2,5 mg): 10 mg x4 am/pm with breakfast, lunch, before training, dinner sublingually used

Mesterolone (Proviron): 25 mg x4 am/pm with breakfast, lunch, before training

Exemestane: 25 mg daily

25mg ephedrine HCL-200mg of caffeine-300mg aspirin before training (ECA stack)

20mcg clenbuterol HCL & 20mcg with lunch

Spironolactone-Furosemide per os (optional)

It should be clarified that, mentioning dosages is something _officially unapproved medically_, for various different reasons:

1) These drugs are created for therapeutic purposes, in order to treat specific diseases.

2) The medical recommended dosage is almost 1/10, that athletes use for muscle anabolism. Physicians who prescribe AAS have the specialty of pathology, endocrinology, and surgery.

3) Each steroid user has his personal goals; therefore his steroid abuse is modified according to his subjective targets. Some wish to be casual recreational gym rats and amateur athletes, while others want to get into competitive national contests. Therefore everyone will take different risks, based on his

personal plan. The fact that I was myself quite abusive does not mean in any way that I suggestand recommend my abusive cycles.

4) For certain drugs there are specific protocols. For example, somatropin is known to work as fat burning agent under small dose, while at larger it leads to muscle development and growth.

Similarly, if insulin overcomes a specific dosage depending on the weight of the athlete, runs the risk of hypoglycemic coma. Therefore we suggest the use of 1 IU/kg of bw, along with 1gr of carbs per kg of bw (100 kg/220 lbs = 10 IU: 5 IU am/pm plus 50 gr+50gr carbs am/pm).

CNS stimulants are also risky, as well as diuretics.

They can easily become lethal medications in a blink of an eye.

These cycles are not intended to be used for healthy people, nor are intended to treat diseases. Note that the medical community does not use of PEDs, for non-medical purposes (Hippocrates law).

However, in the form that our sport has evolved, the contribution of medical science is somethinginevitable. Drugs have side effects whether used in large dosages, or small and prolonged.

Bodybuilding

LABORATORY TESTS – MONITORING THE PROFIL OF THE ATHLETE

Before the beginning of a cycle, it is necessary for the steroid user, to undergo specific laboratory tests, in order to evaluate his general health condition. Adverse effects and possible tissue damage is dependent on various parameters, such as age, time and dosage of abuse, combination of PED's, life style, proper nutrition, medical prevention rules, proper supplementation and family history. Dislipidemia, transaminemia and erythrocytosis are among the commonest distortions, which should inhibit an alleged user from starting a cycle. Otherwise, during the course of a cycle things may get even worse and perhaps the user will be forced to cease the cycle. Occasionally, symptoms appear that justify a bad shape (pain under the right costal arch, jaundice, epistaxis, chest pain, gynecomastia, edema, headache, foggy mind, blurred vision).

- HEMATOLOGIC ASSESSMENT: Hematocrit, Hemoglobin, Platelets, Iron, Ferritin and Cobalamine(B12)

-RENAL ASSESSMENT: Urea, Creatinine, Uric acid, 24h creatinine urine clearance, **glomerular filtration rate**(GFR) and urine microscopic analysis

-HEPATIC ASSESSMENT: SGOT/AST, SGPT/ALT, γGT, ALP, Total Bilirubin (Direct/indirect), LDH

-CARDIOVASCULAR ASSESSMENT: HDL, LDL, TC, Triglycerides, Homocysteine

-TUMOR MARKERS: PSA, AFP, CEA, CA 19.9

-THYROID ASSESSMENT: TSH, T3, T4, FT3, FT4, Anti-TPO, Anti-TG, U/S

-COAGULATION ASSESSMENT: INR, APTT, Fibrinogen

A typical cardiovascular check up includes:
- Frontal X-ray of the thoracic cavity, that reveals the shape of the heart (front image) and assessment of the cardiothoracic index.

- ECG, that reveals any recent or former AMI (acute myocardial infarction), arrhythmias (ventricular or atrial), LVH (left ventricular hypertrophy).

- Echocardiography (Triplex U/S), that illustrates the size and functionality (estimated ejection fraction) of all cardiac chambers, valves, the presence of structural abnormalities in the myocardium.

Furthermore the ascending aorta and aortic arch is illustrated and tested for their morphology and functionality.

Laboratory testing is performed under fasting conditions (eight hour fast), for proper assessment of lipid profile (Triglycerides).Proper hydration for optimal assessment of renal function, while enough hydration also ensures that blood collection becomes easier; especially in cases of erythrocytosis (increased blood viscosity).

=>Possible causes of elevated values:

- HEMATOCRIT: anabolic androgenic steroids (AAS), dehydration, smoking, living at high altitude (>2000 m)

- UREA: poor hydration, increased intake of animal protein (nitrogen retention-azothemia)

- CREATININE: rhabdomyolysis (CPK>1000), increased creatine intake (>10gr/day), daily red meat consumption, non-steroidal anti-inflammatory drugs (NSAID's), increase muscle mass (BMI>30)

- SGOT/AST, SGPT/ALT: 17 alkylated per os AAS, rhabdomyolysis, paracetamol, alcohol abuse, Non Alcoholic Fat Liver Disease (NAFLD)

- GGT, ALP: alcohol abuse, liver disease involving cholestasis and jaundice (biliary duct occlusion)

- LDL, TC: trans & SFAs, refined sugar, lack of EFAs (LA, OA, ALA, CLA, GLA, DHA, EPA)

- TRIG: fish oil (DHA & EPA) deficiency

- BILIRUBIN: cholestasis, jaundice, liver disease

- CPK: rhabdomyolysis, muscle catabolism, viral infection (EBV), acute myocardial infarction (AMI), cocaine abuse

- INR: AAS abuse

- UA: increased intake of animal proteins, involved in purine's metabolism, uric arthritis- gout

- B12: DECREASE equals to megaloblastic anemia (cyanocobalamine deficiency) (MCV>100), as a result of either malnutrition, or alcoholism

- TSH: Hypothyroidism, Hashimoto hypo

- Fe: hemosiderosis-hemochromatosis (iron intoxication), hemolytic anemia, inflammation of the liver (hepatitis), or liver tissue death

- Ca 19.9: Visceral inflammation (liver-bile, pancreas, stomach, small and large intestine-bowel)

- CEA: general tumor marker, lungs

- AFP: testicular seminoma

- PSA: benign prostate hypertrophy (BPH), prostatitis, prostate cancer

- CRP: inflammation

-ESR: inflammation

LABORATORY ASSESSMENT DURING PHYSICAL STRESS

During vigorous physical activity, either indoors anaerobic at the gym, or outdoors aerobic, specific biochemical and hormonal evaluations are distorted.

Contractile muscles undergo rupture; in other words, muscle fibers are torn and myoblobin is released into the blood stream. This protein carries oxygen to skeletal muscles, in similar way hemoglobin does to the rest of tissues. Myoglobin is a nephrotoxic substance to renal glomeruli, thus serum creatinine (CRE) is elevated.Creatine kinase (CPK) enzyme increases up to ten fold. Potassium (K) the main intracellular element is released in the bloodstream. When its concentration reaches high levels, myocardium undergoes arrythmia, such as atrial fibrillation and ventricular tachycardia.Striated muscle rupture equals to cellular death, therefore lactate dehydrogenase (LDH) elevates too.Dehydration will lead to a higher osmolality of plasma.In other words, plasma gets more concentrated and serum urea (BUN) elevates.

White blood cells initially increase, since exercise is a form of inflammatory process. However, when overtraining occurs, the antiflammatory hormone cortisol is released from adrenal glands. Cortisolemia is linked with an increase of C-reactive protein (CRP), an acute inflammatory marker.Chronic mental and physical stress, such as in marathon, triathlon and cycling, will eventually lead to a cortisol crush, due to adrenal fatigue and insufficiency.During that time the absolute number of leukocytes is lowered and so does immune response.Muscle degradation and catabolism will lead to drop of serum albumen and immunoglobulin levels IgA, IgD, IgG, IgM.

Chronic cortisolemia is associated to hypogonadism and low LH/TT.

Moreover, SHBG increases and FT goes down. This is why chronic fatigue syndrome is combined to a loss in libido.

Electrolytes are lost through sweating, so Na, Cl, Mg, Ca will be remarkably low. The hypocalcemia and hypomagnesemia will cost in muscle spasms, known as cramps.Considering the fact that striated muscles, myocardium and liver posses common receptors for transaminases, its is obvious that Alanine transaminase (ALT) and Aspartic transaminase (AST) will be increased.In order to differentiate from Acute Myocardial Infarction (AMI), we should evaluate the troponin protein that increases within 24 hours of heart attack.In order to differentiate from potential liver disease, we should evaluate the cholestatic enzymes Gama glutamino transferase (γGT) and Alkaline phosphatase (ALP).Lactic acid concentration is also found remarkably high.Serum glucose (GLU) initially drops. Soon after hepatic and muscle glycogen stores get depleted, neoglycogenesis through glucagon and cortisol will restore serum glucose.

In this time period, free fatty acids start to elevate in serum, due to beta oxidation of adipose tissue.Lactic acid concentration elevates, leading to metabolic acidosis, where blood pH lowers and reaches 7.35.

Lungs hyperventilate in order to eliminate carbon dioxide. Through hypocapnia, blood pH becomes alkalized.

Hypomagnesaemia and hypocalcaemia will lead to muscle spasms, the so called cramps.

In conclusion, strenous exercise is characterized as an acute metabolic episode.In cellular level, endorphins drop, leading to moodiness; while cytokines are increased, leading to joint pains.In urine microscopic evaluation, we observe microscopic hematuria and traces of cylinders.

MAIN ADVERSEEFFECTS OF AAS

1. CARDIOVASCULAR SYSTEM:

- Reduction of HDL, increased LDL/TC => atheromatic index distortion (> 5) => increased risk of acute myocardial infarction (AMI)

- Cardiomegaly & Left Ventricular Hypertrophy (larger left ventricular mass, left ventricularindex and interventricular septum thicknesses) => chronic heart failure, hypertension

- Altered endothelial integrity of coronary arteries => spasm, in combination with nicotine => ischemia (angina pectoris), chronic heart disease

- Increased serum levels of sodium, calcium& magnesium=> arrhythmias (atrial/ventricular)

Most frequent causes of cardiovascular mortality in bodybuilders:

1) Heart arrhythmia (ventricular tachycardia) from CNS stimulants abuse, or hyperkalemia (elevated serum potassium), due to spirolactone abuse

2) AMI as a result of poor atheromatic profile, coronary vasoconstriction due to CNS stimulants abuse

3) Hemorrhagic cerebral stroke due to aneurysm rupture as a result of increased systolic blood pressure from CNS stimulants abuse

Bodybuilding

4) Chronic heart failure, as a result of Left Ventricular Hypertrophy, mostly from Somatropin-Somatomedin C abuse (GH/IGF1)

2. LIVER-BILIARY TRACT:

- Pharmaceutical hepatitis: Elevation of liver enzymes-transaminases (SGOT, SGPT/AST, ALT), mainly by 17 alkylated AAS per os (oxandrolone, stanozolone, methadrostenolone, oxymetholone, methyltestosterone, methyltrienolone-M3).

These elevations attributed to the intake of oral steroids are usually asymptomatic, transient and return to baseline levels within several weeks after cessation.

- Cholestasis => obstructive jaundice.

Clinical symptoms include nausea, fatigue, itching followed by dark-brownish urine (elevated **urobilinogen**) and jaundice (yellowing of the eye's sclera, skin-elevated bilirubin).

Jaundice can be prolonged, even if AAS are discontinued.

Serum elevations of cholestatic markers (ALP, GGT, bilirubin-direct/indirect), are present.

GGT is the most distinctive enzyme for the detection of hepatic dysfunction.

The esophagus presents varicose bleeding risk, since the venous plexus is seriously developed (portal hypertension).

- Hepatic peliosis (hemorrhagic cysts in hepatic lobes) => structural changes => severe liver dysfunction.

This rare syndrome is potentially reversible, under the discontinuation of AAS. Otherwise hepatic rupture =>sudden abdominal pain and severe internal bleeding=>haemoperitoneum and vascular collapse-Hepatocellular carcinoma, where liver transplantation is the only available therapy of choice for selected patients without the possibility of extrahepatic metastasis.

It should be noted that, during the autopsy of Andreas Munzer in 1996, multiple tumors of walnut size were found on the surface of his liver.

HEPATOPROTECTIVE SUPPLEMENTS

The anabolic androgenic steroids (AAS) are highly toxic to the hepatocyte and cause significant damage, both to the structure and function of the hepatic parenchyma.Especially the hepatotoxic 17 alkylated orals, which significantly disrupt the excretory function of the organ.

Alkylation of the steroid molecule ensures that the particular substance will sustain the detoxification process of the liver, right after its entrance through the portal vein.This alkylation stresses the liver and transaminemia occurs (three digit serum values of liver enzymes ALT/AST-SGOT/SGPT>100).

During the period of the precontest preparation, the athlete should abstain from hepatotoxic substances such as ethyl alcohol, paracetamol (acetaminophen), nonsteroidal anti-inflammatory drugs (NSAIDs).Apart from this, he should use hepatoprotective supplements with meals, since supplementation provides medical prevention and ensures that liver enzymes are not that much elevated (20%).

Supplements with hepatoprotective capacity include:

1) The ursodeoxycholic acid (UDCA) is a bile salt that is mainly used in the formula of cholastic liver disorders.It reduces cholesterol in bile and stones, reduces the excretion of cholesterol from the liver cells and reabsorption in the gut.It is

extremely useful in cases of cholestasis, where jaundice occurs. Its use has been found to improve clinical symptoms of jaundice and liver biochemistry as well (decrease ALP, γGT, Bil).

2) The glutathione (GSH) is a tripeptide consisting of three amino acids (glutamine, cysteine, glycine) and is the most powerful antioxidant in nature. It prevents oxidation of red blood cells, helps in detoxification of the liver parenchyma, strengthens the immune system, improves skin quality, brain metabolism and frequently used as an anti-aging agent. Glutathione's action in the liver ensures the removal of the toxic waste products and neutralizes free radicals reactive oxygen compounds and heavy metals. Injectable-parenteral administration of glutathione ensures its direct action, compared to the oral (per os form), where part of it is degradated by the gastric fluid.

3) N-acetyl-cysteine (NAC) is a precursor of glutathione and used to increase the glutathione reserves in the body.

N-acetyl cysteine is also effective in reducing the death rate and preventing the permanent harm caused by paracetamol (acetaminophen) poisoning.

4) The alpha-lipoic acid (alpha lipoic acid) is a potent antioxidant, that has also been shown that restores glutathione and vitamin levels (vitamin E, C).

Therefore, it is a potent agent against free radicals and oxidative stress.

5) Silymarin (silymarin-milk thisle) is a hepatoprotective substance with multiple actions.

It stabilizes the membrane of liver cells by preventing the entry of toxins into the body. It increases cell regeneration in the liver and stimulates the synthesis of proteins. This results in increasing the production of new liver cells replace the old damaged.It helps prevent the depletion of glutathione in liver cells.Finally, it promotes the flow of bile from the liver to the intestine, which then cleaves the fats from food. Silymarin is used in several of the stages of liver disease by AAS as in pharmaceutical hepatitis in fatty infiltration of the liver and cirrhosis. It does not offer substantially though, in cases of cholestasis.

6) Liv-52 is a mixture of herbal preparation (Basma, Tamarix gallica, herbal extracts of Capparis spinosa, Cichorium intybus, Solanum nigrum, Terminalia arjuna and Achillea millefolium).It is effective in cases of drug hepatitis, non alcoholic fatty liver disease, and cirrhosis. It protects the hepatic parenchyma and promoting the regeneration of liver cells.The protective effect of Liv-52 can be attributed to its diuretic effect too.

7) Finally, lipotropic substances choline-inositol-lecithin, that prevent excessive accumulation of fat in the liver and help nonalcoholic fatty liver disease (NAFLD).

3. URINARY SYSTEM (KIDNEYS):

AAS have a direct toxic effect on glomeruli => elevation of urea (> 80mg/dl), creatinine (> 1.5mg/ dl) => azotemia, uremia => mild renal insufficiency.

Protein and creatine supplements with a high protein intake of >300 g/day increase glomerular filtration rates (GFR) and are associated with focal segmental glomerulosclerosis (FSG) and acute tubular necrosis (ATN).During precontest preparation & glycogen depletion phase, the high consumption of animal protein (>3gr/kg), leadsto ammoniaimia (skin and sweat get a characteristic heavy odor of ammonia).As known, ammonia is a waste product in urea cycle, being toxic to brain's function (increase in hepatic coma). Ketosomes are detected in a biochemical analysis, as a result of a high protein-low carbohydrate dieting, leading to exhalation of ketones (rotten apple smell).

Excessive over-training causing rhabdomyolysis (CPK>1000),induces microscopic hematuria (pinkish color), the presence of cylinders, that are equal to proteinuria. Under normal circumstances, kidneys don't excrete protein (proteinuria). High protein consumption produces acidic urine (pH<5).That, along with increase of calcium retention (nandrolone abuse),could lead to kidney stones formation.

Kidney tumors (Wilm's tumor or nephroblastoma) are rare cases of cancer. However we have to realize that kidneys are directly affected by AAS excretion, especially trenbolone, which gives characteristic brown color urine.

Because kidneys contribute to systemic blood pressure (renin-angiotensin, aldosterone), CNS stimulants can lead to proximal and distal tubular necrosis. Diuretics also have a negative impact on renal function, particularly when it's accompanied by water restriction (dehydration).

4. REPRODUCTIVE SYSTEM (SEX GLANDS)

- Suppression of the HPTA => primary hypogonadism (normal/elevated levels of LH, FSH, low levels of total and free testosterone), which gradually turns into secondary (low levels of total and free testosterone, low levels of FSH, LH) or late onset hypogonadism =>testicular atrophy, reduce in semen production and quality, motility, oligo (<20,000,000 sperm/ml)or azoospermia, changes in libido => infertility

- Gynecomastia (breasttenderness)

- Hypertrophy of the prostate gland (BPH) =>interruption during night sleep for urination (nicturia), difficulty during the start of urination and the leakage of a small amount of urine on the underwear

- Malignant hyperplasia of prostate gland

- Irreversible masculinisation in women (acne, hirsutism, changes in libido, voice deepening, clitoris enlargement, menstrual irregularities and reduction of the breasts)

5. HEMATOPOIETIC AND HAEMOSTATIC SYSTEM:

- Elevation of Hematocrit-Hemoglobin (erythrocytosis effect) => increase in blood viscosity =>epistaxis (nose bleeding), raise in blood pressure and risk for thrombotic stroke => atherosclerosis => rupture of cerebral aneurism

- Prolonged coagulation time (PT, APTT, INR) => inadequate hemostatic ability

6. NEUROLOGICAL - PSYCHIATRIC:

- AAS induced neurotoxicity.

A wide range of psychiatric side effects induced by the use of AAS such as episodes of insomnia, aggression (physical and verbal), irritability, anxiety, neurosis, mood swings-emotional instability, hypomania, manic episodes, depression, bipolar disorder and psychosis (delusions, agitation, ideas of reference, hallucinations, misconceptions)It should be noted that, the profound effects on mental and behavior are correlated to the severity of abuse in terms of dosage and time period, the psychiatric background of the user, his personality and genetic predisposition.

7. IMMUNE SYSTEM:

- At high doses and long-term abuse => disruption of T-lymphocytes of the thymus and spleen => susceptibility to infections.

Nandrolone and oxymethelone abuse trigger the production of pro-inflammatory cytokines (IL-1b/TNF-a).

These cytokines are involved in autoimmune and/or inflammatory diseases.

- Chronic AAS abuse => immunoglobulins (IgG, IgM, IgA, IgD, IgE) **deficiency** and in combination with over training-diet, decrease in white blood cells (WBCs) number.

- AAS abuse crushes on anti-inflammatory (catabolic) cortisol, therefore reducing the strength of the immune system.

8. CARCINOGENESIS:

- Hepatocellular carcinoma and hepatoma
- Malignant hyperplasia of prostate gland
- Nephroblastoma (Wilm's tumor)

MAIN ADVERSE EFFECTS OF NON-AAS PEDs

1) HGH (GROWTH HORMONE-SOMATROPIN):
- acromegaly (arthritis, fatigue fractures)
- diabetes mellitus type II (non insulin dependent), hypothyroidism
- cardiomegaly (chronic abuse) =>increased rate of cardiovascular disease and progressive heart failure
- carpal tunnel syndrome
- obstructive sleep apnea (thickening of the upper airways: pharynx, larynx and glottis) =>hypoventilation and low oxygenation in the brain
- association with colorectal cancer, leukemia, prostate, melanoma (promotion of IGF1 hypersecretion)

2) INSULIN:
- hypoglycemic episode (Slow release insulin)=>cold sweat, chills, cool, pale skin, dry mouth, fast heartbeat, tightness in the chest=> collapsus => coma => death
- lipodystrophy(Long-term use of insulin can cause lipodystrophy at the site of repeated insulin injections. Lipodystrophy includes lipohypertrophy-thickening of adipose tissue-and lipoatrophy-thinning of adipose tissues)

3) DIURETICS:

- hypovolemia and dehydration => hypotension => hypovolemic shock => collapsus

- reduction of all electrolytes and minerals (furosemide) => hypokalemia, hyponatremia, hypocalcemia, hypomagnesemia => muscle spasms/cramps and metabolic alkalosis

- elevation of potassium (hyperkalemia from potassium sparing diuretics) and metabolic acidosis (spironolactone) => severe arrhythmias (ventricular tachycardia, fibrillation) => cardiac arrest

- dose-dependent gynecomastia (abuse of spironolactone).

4) STIMULANTS:

CLENBUTEROL- b2 stimulant with sympathomimetic, adrenergic action.

- cardiac arrhythmias (atrial fibrillation, ventricular tachycardia), palpitations due to the positive inotropic effect on the cardiac muscle => heart attack, cardiac arrest

- angina pectoris (ischemic effect) as a result of coronary vasoconstriction

- direct cardiotoxic effect on the myocardium tissue with necrotic scars

- increased blood pressure => headache, epistaxis, hemorrhagic stroke

- rapid breathing-respiration

- sweating, hand tremors, restlessness and insomnia

- nausea

- hypokalemia (decrease in serum potassium levels) => muscle spasms – cramps.

EPHEDRINE- a & b stimulant receptors with sympathomimetic, adrenergic action.

- sweating, hand tremors, restlessness and hypomania
- severe nausea, vomiting and diarrhea
- increased blood pressure =>headache, epistaxis, hemorrhagic stroke
- cardiac arrhythmias
- hyperpyrexia
- insomnia

CAFFEINE-methylxanthine with stimulant action in the central and autonomous nervous system.

- irritability-restlessness, tremor, sweating, anxiety and panic disorder
- rapid breathing-respiration
- nausea and diarrhea
- cardiac arrhythmias (ventricular tachycardia – fibrillation), precordial chest pain
- increased blood pressure =>headache
- mild form of rebound associated with withdrawal symptoms (fatigue, headache, irritability, depressed mood, inability to concentrate, sleepiness or drowsiness, stomach pain and joint pain)

thyroxine (t4)
- cardiac arrhythmias (tachycardia), heart palpitations

- triggering angina or congestive heart failure
- increased bowel motility
- exophthalmos (eyes bulging)
- insomnia
- sweating, restlessness, irritability, anxiety, sleep disorders
- muscle catabolism and regain of weight, after cessation (typical rebound effect, since BMR drops)

AMPHETAMINES- stimulant with adrenergic action in the myocardium and psychotropic in the central nervous system.

- increased blood pressure=>headache, epistaxis
- hypertensive episode => hemorrhagic stroke due to aneurysm rupture
- nausea, vomiting, diarrhea, weight loss, blurred vision, dry mouth
- erectile dysfunction
- contraction in the urinary bladder sphincter =>difficulty urinating
- cardiac arrhythmias (atrial fibrillation, ventricular tachycardia) =>heart attack, cardiac arrest
- emotional instability, tremors, anxiety, insomnia, hypomania, "amphetamine psychosis "(delusions, paranoia)
- dependence and addiction associated with withdrawal symptoms (anxiety, depressed mood, fatigue, increased appetite, sleep disorders).

5) Recombinant human erythropoietin (-rEPO)

glycoprotein, produced by recombinant DNA technology, that has the same biological activity as the endogenous hormone, which induces erythropoiesis.

- hyperviscosity due to polycythemia => increased peripheral vascular resistance =>thrombotic complications: deep venous thrombosis, pulmonary embolism, stroke

- increased blood pressure =>headache, blurred vision, hypertensive encephalopathy, cerebrovascular accident or myocardial infarction

- association with myeloid malignancies (myelodysplastic syndromes/leukemia (EPO can act as a growth factor for any tumor type, particularly blood malignancies).

MECHANISMS OF DAMAGE BY PEDS USE

CARDIOVASCULAR SYSTEM

The abuse of Performance Enhancing Drugs (PEDs) has been associated with the occurrence of serious cardiovascular events in athletes, including the development of cardiomyopathy, arrhythmias, myocardial infarction, heart failure, hypertension and thrombosis.

<u>Androgenic anabolic steroids (AAS)</u> disturb serum levels of high density lipoprotein (HDL), low density lipoprotein (LDL), lipoprotein A (Lp-A), total cholesterol and triglycerides. Significant reduction of HDL and elevation of LDL and Lp-A increases the risk of atherogenesis (plack formation), leading to atheromatosis and coronary heart disease. The elevation of LDL parallels the decrease of HDL levels. The adverse effect on serum lipids depends on the type of AAS used, the route of administration, combination of drugs, dosage and time of abuse. However, studies have shown that the recovery on serum lipids after AAS cessation is strongly dependent on duration of the AAS abuse rather than the dosage.

Steroids have been also associated with arrhythmias (atrial fibrillation, ventricular fibrillation, tachycardia).One of the reasons is electrolyte imbalance and hypercalcemia in particular, since it has been well established that under supraphysiological dosages, AAS increase electrolytes and minerals absorption (sodium, calcium, phosphorus, magnesium).

AAS users have been demonstrated to show larger left ventricular mass, larger posterior wall and interventricular septum thicknesses. These changes lead to left ventricular hypertrophy, cardiomegaly and increase the risk of chronic heart failure, hypertension and arrhythmias.It should be noted that, the adverse effects in heart structure and function are expected after prolonged AAS abuse.

AAS abuse and especially androgens may increase blood pressure (BP), since they stimulate the production of aldosterone hormone from kidneys. This mineral corticosteroid is responsible for sodium (and water) retention. Some AAS also do aromatise, converted to estrogen, by the aromatase enzyme. Estrogenic activity is linked with bloating and edema. These two mechanisms are linked to hypertension.

AAS influence the hematological system via three main pathways. Firstly, they stimulate erythropoiesis directly by increasing erythroid colony-forming units in the bone marrow and promoting their differentiation into erythropoietin-responsive cells.

Secondly,by promoting erythropoietin (EPO) synthesis in the kidney.

Thirdly, by increasing iron absorption in small intestine, that becomes substrate for hemoglobin protein synthesis. Increased hemopoiesis leads to erythrocytosis and finally polycytemia. The later could become a risk factor for cardiovascular disease, since blood viscosity increases dramatically, as hematocrit elevates.AAS also influence platelet aggregation that results in vascular disease due to enhanced blood-clot formation increasing the risk of cardiovascular events (myocardial infarction, thrombotic stroke, cerebrovascular hemorrhage).AAS prolong bleeding time and sabotage hemostasis. INR, APTT increase and enhance fibrinolysis.This mechanism is contradictive with the platelets aggregation effect.In the bottom line, AAS break down coagulation processing, but on the other hand they induce clot formation, through hematocrit elevation and fibrinogen elevation.

Stimulants with sympathomimetic, adrenergic action elevate heart rate and BP and may exacerbate cardiac arrhythmias (atrial fibrillation, ventricular tachycardia), myocardial ischemia (vasoconstriction) resulting in sever or even fatal cardiovascular complications (heart attack, cardiac arrest). Moreover studies have shown that stimulants such as clenbuterol have a direct cardiotoxic effect on the myocardium tissue with necrotic scars.

The abuse of CNS stimulants such as amphetamines, ephedrine alkaloids, methylxanthines (caffeine) beta2-agonists (clenbuterol-salbutamol) contribute to left ventricular hypertrophy, due to systemic hypertension. Furthermore, their positive inotropic effect on the cardiac muscle increases the risk of cerebrovascular hemorrhage.

Somatropin's (hGH) prolonged abuse of increases permanently the size of internal organs, through IGF1 effect in tissues. Effect on myocardial growth is evident, leading to cardiomegaly, increased rate of cardiovascular disease and progressive heart failure (Greg Kovacs 2013 RIP).The enlarged heart muscle has greater oxygen demands, which under certain circumstances can lead to ischemic events.

The excess of GH and IGF-I causes a specific derangement of cardiomyocytes, leading to abnormalities in cardiac muscle structure and function, inducing a specific cardiomyopathy. This is characterized by concentric cardiac hypertrophy, diastolic dysfunction and eventually impaired systolic function leading to heart failure. The coexistence of hypertension and diabetes may further aggravate cardiomyopathy. It should be noted that, when Florence Griffith-Joyner (Flo Jo) died at the age of 38 years, her heart was enlarged consistent with this specific cardiomyopathy.

Recombinanthuman erythropoietin (rEPO) induces erythropoiesis.Erythrocythemia enhances hyperviscosity and increases the risk for thrombotic complications such as myocardial infarction, pulmonary embolism and cerebrovascular stroke. Another possible pathogenetic mechanism for the adverse cardiovascular effects of rEPO's abuse is the increased blood pressure due to erythrocythemia.

AAS - INDUCED HYPERTENSION

Bodybuilders abuse androgens that make kidneys to release EPO.

As a result hemopoiesis will elevate hemoglobin and hematoctrite.Thus, blood's viscosity increases and blood becomes thicker. This is a serious factor for ischemic stroke,because it can lead to occlusion of cerebral arteries. This occurs even more easily, especially if athlete smokes. Nicotine is known to promote platelets aggregation.

Moreover, bodybuilders abuse CNS stimulants in order to enhance beta oxidation of adipose tissue. Ephedrine & Clenbuterol HCL, thyroxine and triodothyronine, amphetamines and caffeine are among them. These adrenergic sympatheticomimetic substances elevate systemic blood pressure dramatically, both systolic and diastolic.As a result, a cerebral aneurism is highly likely to occur, under stressing circumstances, such as squats or HIIT.Ischemic strokes have usually better prognosis, rather than hemorrhagic strokes.In hemorrhagic stroke,the area where blood is spread into cerebral cortex,is destroyed and equals with cellular death.Hemorage compresses cortex and edema takes place.

Another factor that elevates blood pressure is aldosterone hormone.
As we know,AAS promote water retention,known as edema into the muscle.This is the result of sodium retention, the main extracellular element.

AAS that aromatize lead to water retention as well.Estrogens are linked with this edema and puffy look.Therefore a bodybuilder under off season, who abuses steroids that aromatise,has greater chances of developing hypertension.

As preventing rules, the use of salicylic acid will inhibit platelets agreggation.A diet low in sodium also helps, while blood donation lowers bloods volume.

AAS induce thromboembolism, through another mechanism.

Fibrinogen is a clotting factor elevated under steroid abuse. Thus, blood is more likely to form clots and embolism.Tobacco also promotes thrombosis, throughnicotine. This substance is known to disrupt the endothelium of arteries, leading to platelets aggregation.

However, few AAS that don'taromatise are capable to increase BP (Patrick Arnold). Flyoxymesterone and trenbolone are among them.

Both of them suppress the catabolic glucocorticosteroid cortisol (this is the reason of their high anabolic effect).But they also suppress the mineral corticosteroid aldosterone.So this is the reason they have zero water retention (Peter Van Mol).

However, other mechanisms that involve inhibition of the enzyme 11-hydroxylase,will eventually lead to increased blood pressure.Kidneys have this specific enzyme, in order to protect them from increased blood pressure from cortisol.This enzyme converts cortisol into the inactive cortisone (synthetic form).The reason of that is the fact aldosterone's receptors are sometimes bound by cortisol and the problem initiates.

When inhibition of 11 hydroxylase occurs, another corticosteroid deoxycorticosterone is synthesized,leading to increased blood pressure(Nelson Vergel).

EPISTAXIS AMONG BODYBUILDERS

The phenomenon of epistaxis (nosebleeding) is often observed in athletes who are in a cycle.

This may be due to different causes, depending on the medication administered each time:

1) increase of systolic blood pressure affecting the vessels of the nose, caused either from stimulants such as ephedrine hydrochloride (in combination with caffeine), or clenbuterol hydrochloride (in combination with thyroxin)

2) increase of systolic blood pressure from medications increasing sodium and water retention and aromatize (oxymetholone, methantrostenolone, enanthic testosterone)

3) elevation of hematocrit (and hemoglobin-myoglobin) by the use of androgens (boldenone, oxymetholone), that stimulate erythropoietin (EPO) release, increase red bone marrow activity and iron incorporation into the red cells

4) prolonged coagulation time (elevation of PT, APTT, INR) resulting to inadequate hemostatic ability by the use of hepatotoxic 17 alkylated synthetic derivatives-AAS

AAS AND HOMOCYSTEINE

Homocysteine (Hcy) is a sulfur amino acid, which is biosynthesized during the metabolism of methionine to cysteine mainly involving the B complex vitamins.It is a toxic residue of the metabolism, linked to cardiovascular disease, when accumulated.

Hyperhomocysteinemia induces endothelial injury and endothelial dysfunction, increased platelet activation at the site of microvascular injury, leading to the development of atherosclerosis.Elevation of plasma Hcy levels creates a condition called hyperhomocysteinemia (HHcy), which is characterized into three ranges; moderate (16-30 μmol/L), intermediate (31 - 100 μmol/L) and severe (>100 μmol/L) HHcy.

Hyperhomocysteinemia in combination with other factors (hyperlipidemia, hypertension, smoking, unhealthy diet, stress) promote atherogenesis, atheromatosis and atherosclerosis, that eventually lead to coronary artery disease, peripheral artery disease, stroke, or venous thrombosis.

Recent studies have shown that, a 25% elevation (about 3 μmol/L) of homocysteine's levels is associated with a 10% higher risk of cardiovascular events and a 20% higher risk of stroke. When these concentrations exceed 15 μm/l, there is a 25% increase in mortality. Furthermore, homocysteine is a significant, independent risk factor for Alzheimer's disease, Parkinson's disease and metabolic syndrome.

Anabolic-androgenic steroid (AAS) use has long term effects on plasma concentrations ofhomocysteine. Elevation of homocysteine levels depends on:

a) the type of the AAS:

The 17 alkylated AAS are hepatotoxic and disrupt the metabolism of Hcy in the liver. Those that aromatize (methyldrostenolone, oxymetholone?) increase estrogen (E2) concentration and reduce levels of cobalamine (vitamin B12) and folate. Deficiencies in plasma folate and B12 have been shown to lead to elevated Hcy concentrations.

b) the duration of use:

There is a significant linear relationship between long term AAS abuse and hyperhomocysteinemia.Administration> 6 months leads to an increase of plasma levelsof Hcy.

c) the dosage of AAS

Studies have shown acute hyperhomocysteinaemia in bodybuilders using supraphysiological doses of various AAS preparations.

d) the simultaneous use-stacking of several different AAS

The mechanism of hyperhomocysteinemia during or after AAS abuse is multifactorial. AAS are known to cause marked dyslipidemia, with significant reduction in high density lipoprotein (HDL) and an increase of low density lipoprotein (LDL) increasing the susceptibility to cardiovascular events.Moreover, AAS affect the haemostatic system, through an increased fibrinolytic activity and simultaneously platelet aggregation.

The activation of the coagulation cascade leads to prolonged bleeding time (INR, PT are remarkably elevated). AAS influence the hematological system leading to erythocytosis, by stimulating bone marrow and by promoting erythropoietin synthesis in the kidney.Erythocytosis is associated with blood viscosity, thus coronary, peripheral artery and venous thrombosis.

Synthesis of homocysteine occurs in erythrocytes, thus their higher number contributes to homocysteinemia.

To addresshyperhomocysteinemia, the AAS user should use vitamin B12, folate and betaine (trimethylglycine) supplementation.Moreover, he should avoid alcohol consumption and all other factors that damage the vascular endothelium such as smoking, hypertension, dyslipidemia.

It should be noted that, although the the AAS cessation leads to reduced homocysteine levels, the damage of the vascular endothelium is irreversible.

GENITOURINARY SYSTEM

The intake of androgenic anabolic steroids (AAS) burdens the kidneys through the process of glomerular filtration in the renal parenchyma. The first stage of AAS metabolism takes place into the liver, but later chemicals pass through the glomerulus and renal tubules (proximal & distal) to be excreted. The creatinine serum level, which is a reliable indicator of renal function, increases (> 1.5mg/ dl), as well as urea (>80 mg/ dl) and uric acid (>7.5 mg/ dl). It should be noted that, all these biochemical parameters are affected from several other non-renal factors (state of hydration, vegan diet) and their levels will not be raised above the normal range, until 60% of total kidney function is lost. So, the most reliable indicator of renal function is the measurement of creatinine clearance (GFR) at 24hrs.

Trenbolone is highly nephrotoxic, gives a characteristic brown color urine and should not be combined with other aggravating substances for the kidney, such as non-steroidal anti-inflammatory drugs-NSAID's (diclophenac, nimesulid), antibiotics (aminoglycosides) and diuretics (furosemide).The abuse of trenbolone-stanozolol stacking has been associated with severe cholestasis and acute renal failure (ARF). Findings of renal biopsy reveal a direct toxic effect on glomeruli and renal tubules resulting in focal segmental glomerulosclerosis, tubular necrosis, nephrotic syndrome and eventually ARF.Clinically, the patient presents with edema in the face and lower extremities (from proteinuria, hypoalbuminemia), hypertension, oliguria or even anuria (urine volume<500ml/24h).In microscopic urinalysisproteinuria, microhematuria and cylinders are present.

Besides AAS abuse, athletes have additional factors that could exert stress on renal function, such as overtraining, creatine monohydrate supplementation, high protein intake, elevated BMI (>30) and dehydration.

- During intense over training, where rhabdomyolysis appears (increased serum CPK**>1000**), damaged muscle fibers release myoglobin, a protein responsible for carrying oxygen to skeletal muscles. This protein is nephrotoxic for renal glomeruli and tubules and may lead to acute tubular necrosis and ARF. Kidney function impairment from rhabdomyolysis presents with a dark color of the urine, microscopic hematuria (pinkish, red color), proteinuria or the presence of cylinders. A dark brownish color of the urine is also a feature of liver/ biliary disease, as a result of cholestasis from AAS abuse. This pigmentation is due to urobilirogen, coming from excess conjugated bilirubin (bilirubinuria).

- The use of creatine monohydrate in the form of a supplement, or through the consumption of red meat (high protein intake of >300 g/day) increase glomerular filtration rates and is associated with focal segmental glomerulosclerosis and acute tubular necrosis. Creatine monohydrate with loading doses of 20 g/day for 5 days and then maintenance doses of 5 g/day are considered to be safe, always with proper hydration.

During pre-contest preparation and glycogen depletion phase, the high consumption of animal protein (>3gr/kg), increases serum levels of ammonia (ammonemia), which is a waste product in urea cycle. Ammonia (NH_3) gives skin and sweat a characteristic heavy odor and is toxic to brain's function (hepatic encephalopathy). Moreover, high protein consumption produces acidic (<5.5) urine pH, while vegetarian diet with increased fruits and vegetables result in an alkaline (> 7.5) urine pH. That, along with increase of calcium retention (nandrolone abuse), could lead to hypercalcemia and formation of kidney stones. Nephrolithiasis can cause direct injury to the kidney and plugging of the ureters, especially under dehydration state (urine specific weight >1030). Protein consumption tends to be diuretic, in the absence of carbohydrates and in such cases ketosomes are detected in a biochemical analysis, leading to exhalation of ketones (rotten apple smell).

- Greater body mass (BMI> 30) leads to higher glomerular hyper-filtration, which in time leads to mechanical strain and scarring.Furthermore, studies have found that chronic hyperfiltration from a high-protein diet may accelerate progression to glomerulosclerosis.

In rare cases, abuse of AAS has been associated with the development of kidney tumors (Wilm's tumor or nephroblastoma).

It is well known that, kidneys regulate arterial blood pressure through renin-angiotensin-aldosterone system. Abuse of CNS stimulants such as beta-agonists (clenbuterol) or ephedrine leads to vasoconstriction of renal vessels, chronic systemic hypertension, proximal and distal tubular necrosis and acceleration of renal failure. Diuretics also have a negative impact on renal function, particularly when their abuse is accompanied by water restriction.

The abuse of performance-enhancing drugs (PED's) adversely affects renal function through direct and indirect mechanisms.Firstly, AAS are nephrotoxic and associated with the development of focal segmental glomerulosclerosis and tubular necrosis. On the other hand, rhabdomyolysis, high protein and creatine intake, nephrolithiasis, inadequate hydration and high incidence of polypharmacy are other factors that contribute to a rapid decline in renal function.

HEMATOPOIETIC SYSTEM

The chronic abuse of anabolic androgenic steroids (AAS) leads to increased hematopoiesis in the bone marrow. Certain drugs such as Boldenone, Oxymetholone, Testosterone and Erythropoietin (rEPO) can improve erythropoiesis process and increase hemoglobin, hematocrit.Androgenic-anabolic steroids (AAS) in general stimulate EPO production from renal cortex, production of red cells from bone marrowand enhance iron absorption from the small intestine (jejunum-ileum). Oxymetholone (Anadrol 50) for instance, was medically prescribed to treat severe congenital aplastic anemia, before the discovery of synthetic EPO (r-EPO). Moreover, secondary severe anemia (aplastic, hypoplastic or from organic causes such as chronic renal failure) was treated by the administration of Oxymetholone. AAS have been shown to increase plasma EPO levels in anephric patients and play an important role in the treatment of anemia of end-stage renal disease. AAS may also be more cost-effective than r-EPO and have an advantage of providing anabolic effect. The medical protocol for anemic patient is 1mg/kg of body weight for 3-6 months in order to promote hemoglobin synthesis in bone marrow.Oxymetholone when used for recreational purposes dramatically enhances erythrocytosis resulting in polycythemia.

As hemoglobin rises (Hgb> 18), hematocrit follows an excessive increase about three fold(Htc> 54%), leads to increased blood viscosity and predisposes for thrombotic stroke, pulmonary embolism, hypertension (> 140/90 mmHg) and left ventricular hypertrophy.

Clinical findings and symptoms of erythrocytosis include hot flashes, sweating, flushing of the face and palms, easy bleeding, itching especially after a hot shower (post-bath pruritus), headache, double vision, dizziness. In rare cases, when polycythemia is prolonged, the heart pumps blood harder, which might lead to heart failure.

The use of salicylic acid (aspirin),fish oil (EPA/DHA) and blood donations, or therapeutic phlemotomies are preventing methods.Polyunsaturated fatty acids (PUFAs) have anti-thrombotic activity via suppression of prostaglandins (PGs), which are inflammatory cytokines.Also Aspirin has a thrombolytic-antiplatelet action, against blood coagulationand its use on a daily basis with meals is required. The drug belongs to Non Steroid Anti iflammatory Drugs (NSAIDs),that inhibit PGs, through Thromboxanes (TX) & cycloxygenase enzymes (COX1, COX2). This has a direct effect on the functionality and not their absolute number of platelets.For those who have G6PD enzyme deficiency and cannot use aspirin, the use of fish oil (DHA/EPA), is an alternative choice.

Blood donation is a process that should be performed at regular intervals of three to four months.RBCs life span is of 120 days,therefore a more frequent blood donation/phlebotomy, would stimulate red bone marrow for further production of erythrocytes. One unit of blood drop equals to 330ml.This will lower hematoctit by 3% and hemoglobin of one unit. Too many blood donations will eventually lead to iron deficiency and lowering of ferritin protein (iron stores).

The hematocrit value (Htc) is affected by the state of hydration of the body. Dehydration is followed by more concentrated plasma and falsely (pseudoerythrocytosis) elevated hematoctit-not hemoglobin. That's why hemoglobin is a more reliable evaluation of anemia/polycythemia. Conversely, fluid overload will falsely lead to diluted urine. In that case hematocrit drops and the ratio between hematocrit vs. hemoglobin becomes lower instead of the 3/1 ratio.Serum urea can also confirm that, since it's directly affected by hydration state. The so called water intoxication is a critical condition of over hydration (glycogen depletion phase before a show),where hyponatremia occurs.Under such circumstances,headaches due to cerebral edema are a fact.Confusion,lethargy and fogginess are common symptoms as well.Smoking also increases the hematocrit value by another mechanism, hypoxemia through the production of carbon monoxide (CO), leading as a result to secretion of erythropoietin by the kidney.

The elevated hematocrit of a steroid abuser and a smoker leads to an increased risk of myocardial infarction, since nicotine induces platelet aggregation and occlusive stroke. Moreover, smoking elevates fibrinogen, thus inducing clotting process. Furthermore, it is known that increased hematocrit increases viscosity of the blood-viscosity and makes it more viscous.

Quite often, nose bleeding is observed in athletes who are on steroid cycle. This can be the result of different causes, such as:

1) increase in systolic blood pressure that is caused by CNS stimulants(ECA stack, clenbuterol HCL)

2) increase in systolic blood pressure from AAS abuse (aldosterone secretion),or adrenergic effect of CNS stimulants,

3) elevated hematocrit, resulting to a larger volume of RBCs,

4) coagulopathy (clotting factors PT, APTT, INR distortion) resulting to prolonged bleeding, due to 17 alkylated hepatotoxic AAS

One reason why the use of aspirin is necessary is the fact that anabolic substances increase the platelet aggregation (coagulation components) especially when coexisting with smoking, since nicotine negatively predisposes to this phenomenon. The AAS cause increased thrombin which in turn increases the fibrinogen and therefore promotes clotting.

MUSCLE GROWTH AND CANCER

There is a belief that muscle growth deals with the tumor process and growth.Muscle development involves inflammatory process, such as the cytokines prostaglandins.Hormones as insulin, insulin like growth factor and mTOR as necessary for anabolism.

However,ripampicin has been associated with cancer growth.Same as with IGF1 that promotes tissue growth and hyperplastic phenomena.

Somatomedin C is released from liver under exogenous use of Somatropin.Also under high caloric intake when insulin is released from pancreas, liver also releases insulin growth factor.It is remarkable that the opposite process occurs under fasting and AMPK elevation.

IGF1, insulin and mTOR lower and muscle growth is hindered.Without calories muscles shrink and AMPK protein elevates, linked to longevity.

Metformin is also known to induce this and is speculated to be a preventing drug against cancer.Metformin lowers glycemia and proteins glycosilation,but is also considered as anti aging medication.Metformin is also alternatively used to insulin from bodybuilders who abuse growth hormone.As known GH is diabetogenic and leads to insulin resistance and DM2.

PREVENTION OF SIDE-EFFECTS OF PEDS USE

LIFESTYLE PREVENTIVE TIPS ALONG WITH PEDS USE

- Using supplements and dairy products with phytosterols (plant based estrogens)

- Avoidance of excessive saturated fat and trans fat/refined carbohydrates-sugars

- Regular use of coenzyme Q10, which has the ability to increase aerobic energy production of myocardium, along with magnesium, acting as a mild anti-arrhythmic agent

- Use hepatoprotective supplements (Liv 52, silimarin-milk thisle, glutathione, N-Acetyl cysteine)

- Daily intake of Omega 369 fatty acids, niacin (B3), lecithin, for better atheromatic profile

- Consumption of antioxidants during PCT.

- Use of statins after PCT is through, if necessary.
Note that statins are hepatoxic, diabetogenic and lower Q10 of heart muscle

- Use of salicylic acid-aspirin, through the whole course of androgenic anabolic steroids (AAS) cycle; preferable with breakfast (not post workout)

- Proper hydration (3lt/day, in order urine color to be as clear as possible) and avoidance of diuretics that forces kidneys to overload

- Use of ascorbate-vitamin C during winter, when there is susceptibility to viral infections

- Avoidance of alcohol and hepatotoxic painkillers (paracetamol), non steroid anti-inflammatory drugs (NSAIDs)

- Moderate dosages and avoidance of excessive stacking; not abused over eight weeks

- Preference in prescribed pharmaceuticals and afterwards in legit-reliable underground drugs

- Avoidance of the 17 alkalized hepatotoxic pills and injectables; preferably to be used sublingually

- Daily cardiorespiratory aerobic physical activity

- For acne spots on the back, shoulders and face local use of azelaic acid cream and antibiotic clindamycin lotion.

Hygiene rules with antibacterial soap, while disinfection with pure alcohol 95' is particularly effective.

Also use of ultraviolet radiation is quite effective against sebum production.

HOW PRO'S CYCLE AAS

In professional bodybuilding there is a certain plan-strategy of cycling.So the professional athletes follow two main directions.

The first one, during off season period, is the use of the three main anabolic hormones (testosterone, somatropin, insulin) in moderate doses (maintenance phase). Afterwards, when they are about to start their precontest preparation, they increase doses but also use the variety of anabolics and androgenic steroids.This method serves prevention and maintenance of a good lipid profile and preserves cardiovascular health.

The other concept is the modification of cycling AAS, depending on the particular time period, in combination with diet and training. Cycles have the form of pyramid with progressive elevation of doses, until they reach the peak in the middle of the cycle's progress. Afterwards, they decline until they reach a minimum level. The disadvantage of this method is the possibility of intramuscular abscess formation. This is due to the great amount of gear injected intramuscularly (buttocks, delts). Therefore,estrogenic highly aromatised AAS are preferably used during off season, while non-estrogenic and potent androgens are used during the cutting phase.

Some ambitious bodybuilders take advantage of the hormonal enviroment they have being through the cutting phase.They shift immediately right after a show,switching the cutting non aromatised AAS into the bulking aromatised ones.

Of course, this is supported from a dramatic change in nutrition and training style.Calories and carbs elevate, and almost double so that anabolism is ensured through insulin's rush.

This rebound strategy provides gains in a physique that has being already lean and muscular,as it was the time of the contest.Therefore it is easier to experience the bloating effect that ripped muscle get.

Bodybuilders are practical people, meaning, they are more concerned about musculoskeletal injuries, which will immerse them from training, rather than their internal organs health, which reflect on laboratory tests. They hope and believe that, they will get improved soon after their retirement.

EXERCISE INDUCED CARDIAC REMODELING

The athlete's heart is a deviation of a normal shaped myocardium.It is a natural response, a physiological remodeling to the continuous stimulus of strenuous physical activity, such as endurance running under high intensity.

Many studies have shown that cardiac adjustment varies, depending on the type of training (dynamic or static) and the type of sport. It appears that more than three hours of exercise is required per week to observe adaptive changes, such as the reduction in heart rate and increase in mass of the left ventricle (LV).

Marathon and triathlon runners develop a "drop heart" shape, with enlarged ventricles and thin ventricular walls. This helps hemodynamically-functionally providing a greater ejection fraction (EF) and stroke volume (the ability of the heart muscle to pump blood and the volume of blood in each pulse).On the other hand, exercising with weights-resistance training, in combination with chemical enhancement with Performance Enhancing Drugs (PED's) leads to specific hemodynamic changes in the heart. In particular, increase in heart rate, decrease in stroke volume and ejection fraction (EF).

The LV becomes adapted to these hemodynamic changes, resulting in thickening of the wall with smaller ventricular cavities. Heart is a muscle that is mixed, under histological evaluation; meaning it possesses cardiac muscle fibers and skeletal-striated-contractile muscle fibers.Obviously, this explains how heart becomes enlarged, just by lifting weights. Moreover, androgenic receptors are present in a variety of organs and tissues, such as the heart muscle.Therefore, heart will also react positively, under anabolic-androgenic steroid (AAS) abuse.

The athletic heart differs from the heart of non-athletes, provided that the exercise has a sufficient intensity and duration. Depending on the type of exercise and the kind of sport, we observe an increase of thickening in the LV, especially in dynamic events, such as explosive sports: shot put, sprinting, weight lifting, bodybuilding, powerlifting. An enlarged myocardium, either by aerobic exercise (marathon) or bodybuilding using AAS-HGH/IGF1 has increased requirements for oxygen consumption. Intensive and prolonged anaerobic exercise affects the chamber size, the muscle mass of the LV and the wall thickness of the heart, resulting in an enlarged heart with thick ventricular walls and **interventricular**septum. Ventricular capacity-volume is indirectly proportional to ventricular walls thickening. Consequently, there is the less adequate amount of blood pumped, EF lowers and generally, EF is lower in athletes with large BMI. The hypertrophic myocardium has much greater oxygen needs than usual, so ischemia is more likely to develop, under hypoxic conditions.

On the other hand, a prolonged dynamic physical activity such as aerobic training leads to physiologic hypertrophy of the heart that affects all four chambers with normal or reduced peripheral vascular resistance and with a lower heart rate of the average individual (<60beats/min).

With a larger left ventricle, the heart rate can decrease and still maintain a level of cardiac output necessary for the body. This is an economy of energy myocardium does, since there is no need for faster heart beating.

Therefore, heart beats slower, in order to pump the same amount of blood. Eventually, this reflects directly into a supreme physical condition and a cardiovascular capacity too.

Bodybuilding

The heart of an endurance athlete (marathon runner, cyclist, triathlon) has a characteristic shape on a chest X-ray, "drop shaped" heart with an increased left ventricle (cardio-thoracic index enlarged).

HIIT is a mixed type of aerobic/anaerobic cardio respiratory physical activity. It's beneficial as it saves time, preventing catabolism through specific hormonal signal. It boosts testosterone and growth hormone by lactate production, while it prevents cortisol to elevate significantly. A steroid user, who smokes, avoids cardiovascular aerobic physical activity and consumes saturated-trans fat, develops poor physical condition, with inadequate collateral circulation, high blood pressure and is more likely to develop coronary heart disease, due to atherosclerosis. VO2max and cardio respiratory capacity are significantly dropped.

Cardio at a moderate pace of 60% of VO2max-MRH mostly establishes the collateral circulation and elevates serum levels of high density lipoprotein (HDL). Performing cardio at 80% of VO2max-MHR improves physical condition and cardio respiratory capacity. However that kind of intensity will lead eventually to the development of the athlete's heart.

THE IMPORTANCE OF EXERCISE IN COMPARISON TO STATINES, REGARDING PREVENTION AND TREATMENT OF CARDIOVASCULAR EPISODES

New studies come to reinforce the idea that, regular physical activity is particularly a powerful preventive and therapeutic measure, for the treatment of heart and vascular events.The fact that exercise and proper diet are the best preventing methods, is something well known from the ancient time of Hippocrates.Studies have shown that physical condition and cardiorespiratory capacity, was increased by 10%, under regular aerobic exercise in 12weeks.However,for those patients who were using statins at the dose of 40mg, the increase was just 1.5%.Muscle biopsy revealed at cellular level, that mitochondria's metabolism (powerhouses responsible for energy production) in muscle cells, was increased by 13% for those who trained,while those who exercised but used statins too decreased by 4.5%.

Statins are responsible for lowering dramatically Q10 levels in myocardium.Also a recent study published in JAMA, concluded that musculoskeletal disorders such as arthritis, injuries, and musculoskeletal pains are more frequent in statin users, especially when they are physically active.

Studies have shown that statins significantly increase muscle injury in the exercise, as well as reduce the exercise capacity in animals.Rhabdomyolysis effect is a common biochemical symptom (CPK>1000).The even more impressive is that those who did exercise (walking or cycling) and were not under statinsuse, had a 50% lower mortality than those who were taking statins but not exercised.

Large doses of statins,given under prolonged timing, increase the risk for insulin resistance.Moreover,transaminemia is frequently observed (ALT/SGPT, AST/SGOT). Statins have really proven their value is in patients with coronary heart disease and particularly after acute myocardial infarction, due to the anti-inflammatory action in the vessels. However, they should not be used as drugs just to lower serum cholesterol levels and treat dislipidemia. They are obligatory only under established coronary heart disease.

ANDROGEN EMOTIONAL TOXICITY SYNDROME

The speculated "roid rage" deals with the consequences of performance enhancing drugs (PED's) & androgenic anabolic steroids (AAS) abuse in the mental status and psychology of bodybuilders. The psychopathological aspect of PED's /AAS neurotoxicity and dependence can present as a chronic-long term adverse effect, or in the form of episodes-crisis adverse effect.

Apart from the fact that bodybuilders have an external appearance way freakier that the average individual, the combination of an extreme low carbohydrate, low caloric diet, along with exhausting training along with chemical enhancement abuse, would make an explosive combination, leading eventually to a psychopathologic behavior.

Roid rage has been associated with various psychiatric manifestations such as sleep disorders(insomnia), anxiety, mania, depression, irritability, aggression, violence, suicidal behavior, psychosis, confusion and delirium. It's quite common that heavy steroid users have a lower threshold of patience and lose their temper easier, making them to act spontaneously, driven by their instinct without thinking logically. Long-term abuse may lead to the development of a dependence syndrome and withdrawal symptoms on cessation.

It is well known that brain has androgen receptors (AR) that correspond to different chemical substances, able to cross the blood brain barrier and the placental barrier as well (17 β trenbolone).

As a result, some anabolic steroids with a high level of androgenicity, for instance fluoxymesterone (800 androgenic index) or trenbolone (500 androgenic index), have the ability to bind tighter to the AR. It has being demonstrated that neural junctions transmit signals much faster, reflecting directly to serotonin, dopamine metabolism. However, this is not exclusively linked to the androgenic activity of a particular AAS. Nandrolone decaonate, a 19nortestosterone derivative AAS, prescribed medically for the treatment of osteopenia has been associated with several behavioral disorders in supraphysiological treatment doses (>200mg/15 days).Therefore, on-medical use of AAS carries neurodegenerative potential. Recent animal studies have shown this AAS effect, ranging from neurotrophin unbalance to increased neuronal susceptibility to apoptotic stimuli.

Experimental and animal studies strongly suggest that apoptotic mechanisms are at least in part involved in AAS induced neurotoxicity. Furthermore, a great body of evidence is suggesting that increased cellular oxidative stress to cerebral neurons could play a major role in the pathogenesis of many neurodegenerative disorders, such as manic-depression, or bipolar effect. Several different studies suggest that a wide range of psychiatric side effects induced by the use of AAS is correlated to the severity of abuse in terms of dosage and time period.

In another study, 17β-trenbolone was administered to adult and pregnant rats and the primary hippocampus neurons. Hippocampus is a certain area in the mesencephalon, belonging to the limbic system, associated with behavior. 17β-trenbolone accumulated in adult rat brain, especially in the hippocampus, and in the fetus brain. 17β-trenbolone induced apoptosis of primary hippocampal neurons.Therefore, 17β-trenbolone played critical roles in neurodegeneration. Large doses of trenbolone and bodybuilders-powerlifters-strongmen, which are exposed to 17β-trenbolone by various ways, are all influenced chronically and continually. As a result, it is not only a matter of dose, but duration as well.

Cerebral MRI examinations of persons who abused chronically AAS, showed enlarged the amygdala, a certain area of mesencephalon belonging to the limbic system. Amydgala along with hippocampus determine the emotional status. It's important to mention that metabolism of glutamic acid was also increased. As well known, glutamine is an important amino acid, taking part in brain's metabolism. Moreover, it was demonstrated by psychiatric tests that chronic AAS abusers, suffered from short term amnesia.

Some other anabolic steroids, such as methandrostenolone-methandienone - a methyltestosterone's derivative - aromatize. Aromatization is the production of estrogens, by activation of aromatase enzyme in different tissues (breast, liver, adipose, brain). Estrogens are linked directly with neurotransmitters, such as serotonin, thus improving mood. As a result, dianabol will induce a euphoric effect and addiction is highly to occur, both mentally and physically.

On the other hand testosterone is a natural existing hormone, which males produce on a daily basis. It is not a synthetic derivative like AAS. However, investigations concerning the testosterone's effect in human behavior revealed that increased levels of circulating testosterone in serum was associated with significant increase in anger and hostility. Testosterone undecaonate, enanthate, cypionate are different types of esters used in hormonal replacement therapy (HRT) in males during andropause.

Concerning hypogonadal men, who undergo andropause, testosterone supplementation has beneficial effects on mood, self esteem, and sexual desire. Testosterone replacement therapy (TRT) has positive, beneficial effects on depression, anemia, metabolic syndrome, obesity, sarcopenia, osteopenia and fatigue. It improves insulin resistance, physical strength, libido, bone mineral density and red blood cell count.

Testosterone application has shown that a single administration of 100mg TU in eugonadal males, results in supraphysiological serum testosterone levels, resulting in minor mood changes. On the contrary, hypogonadal males who undergo HRT have no detectable-to limited changes in behavior.

The current literature on AAS usage suggests that some users develop episodes of insomnia, aggression (physical and verbal), irritability, anxiety, neurosis, mood swings-emotional instability, hypomania, manic episodes, depression and rarely phychosis-missconcemptions. However, AAS abusers expose themselves to extreme higher doses, that quite common is referred as stacking cycles of different substances. What is most important, is to evaluate the psychiatric background of those users, being able to identify if they had a poor genetic predisposition and mental illness history, before they even begun AAS use. We conclude that each person reacts different under same circumstances, depending on his character, temper, or level of education. Besides the genetic predisposition of the user the extent of neurotoxicity of PED's/AAS also varies with the duration, dosage of abuse, concurrent organic diseases, use of other medications and neurotoxic chemicals, such a**marijuana**(weed), ethanol or narcotics.

Other drugs that belong to the class of CNS stimulants (ephedrine HCL, clenbuterol HCL, methyloxanthines, amphetamines), as soon as they are discontinued, rebound effect is more likely to occur. It is a similar case to a hangover, resulting from alcohol abuse, or withdrawal symptoms of cocaine. Remarkably, it was narcolepsy to which amphetamines were manufactured. Therefore, we could make the assumption that amphetamines, ephedrine alkaloids, methyloxanthines, or even $\beta 2$ agonists are highly addictive too, when they are ceased abruptly. Another class of narcotics, acting as potent painkillers, has a highly addictive effect on brain's chemistry. Codeine is an opioid, which belongs to the same family with heroin. Nubain (synthetic morphine) was a widely used pain killer among professional athletes and there are rumors that this kind of drug was claimed to be the reason that IFBB Pro, Paul De Mayo was pronounced dead at the age of 38.

PREPARING FOR A SHOW

We assume that the competition is held on Sunday. The previous Saturday the last leg workout should take place, in order the quads and hams to be free of any water retention and edema. Training brings blood and this will lead to excess fluid retention. The last torso workout should be performed on Wednesday, for the same reason; while abs has to be worked out till the last training.

One week prior to the contest, the oily injections have to be withdrawal (drostanolone,trenbolone,methenolone,testosterone propionate) and just keep up with the water based (stanozolol depot, trenbolone base, testosterone suspension). The very last week before the show, we maintain the aromatised free orals (stanozolol,oxandrolone,fluoxymesterone,mesterolone) and of course the aromatase inhibitors (anastrozol,letrozol,exemestane).

Some athletes, who are already ripped and dry, tend to use Oxymetholone.

The reason is

1) when estrogens are too low;oxymetholone does not convert to estrogen (as a DHT derivative).

2) oxymetholone can bring extra stamina and endurance because it boosts erythrocytosis and O2 transport to muscles.

In addition, oxymetholone is a powerful anabolic, androgenic and anticatabolic medication that plays a significant role during the low carb diet.

During the last week of glycogen depletion,CNS stimulants are kept and withdrawal with last workout.

After the brutal last week of the low carb-ketogenic diet, the yummy time of glycogen loading follows. This is perhaps the most crucial moment of the whole preparation. Proper carbohydrate and glycogen loading can be the key to success.

It would be wise to lower to the half the aromatase inhibitors. My belief is that too much of them will eventually hinder glycogen loading. Aromatase inhibitors crush estrogens, meaning technically poor glycogen formation and practically zero water retention.

Water consumption during glycogen depletion phase, has to be at least five liters. Too much of water apparently blocks ADH from kidneys (anti diuretic hormone, or vasopressin). The so-called "water intoxication" often occurs during that time. In their effort to eliminate the byproducts of ketonic diet, they lead to hyper hydration which leads to hyponatremia that results in the hemodilution. In clinical chemistry this is translated to a lower hematocrite (not hemoglobin) and lower serum urea as well.

With this mechanism the body eliminates the excess subcutaneous fluid retention. However this process can lead to cerebral edema, with symptoms of headache, hypotension, nausea, dizziness and occasionally even faint.

The glycogen depletion phase has to be <100gr of starch (preferably potato and rice).

It is noteworthy that baked potato has a higher glycemic index than boiled. Protein source comes mainly from white meat (turkey, chicken, rooster, rabbit) and fish. In case the physique looks kind of flat and ultra ripped, lean red meat (beef-buffalo, ostrich, horse, deer) can be an alternative option. Egg whites (albumin) and whey protein powder (lactalbumin) are excluded, due to their high sodium content. Animal protein intake must be >3g/kg of body weight.

Glycogen depletion phase is accompanied by water low in sodium.

Table salt is gradually discontinued and not abruptly.Otherwise, aldosterone is stimulated, leading to sodium and water retention, as a compensatory mechanism .Nature is smarter than people think and the system always brings a homeostatic balance.The more glycogen muscle lack off, the better will be filled up from glycogen.Insulin sensitivity is sky-high and insulin rebound will ensure glycogen synthase enzyme will do its job fair enough.Carb loading phase usually depends upon the body type (BMI).

Generally 24/72 hours are enough for muscles (and liver) to get full.

During loading phase, protein consumption is of secondary priority.

Therefore, two grams of protein per bodyweight are enough for positive nitrogen balance. Muscles have received huge amounts and besides workouts no longer take place. What is important is that fiber is strictly prohibited.Fiber can bring serious GIT bloating and gas.Therefore, sweet potato and brown rice are excluded and regular potatoes with white rice are best choices.Pasta and bread are not an option, because of their gluten presence.This plant based protein can hold water and smooth the physique, sort of looking high in estrogens.Oats also excluded for the same reason and their fiber content as well.

The first 24 hours of carb loading are the most critical.

As loading phase proceeds, glycogen stores are gradually filled up and insulin sensitivity hits a plateau. Sodium and water intake are necessary the very first day of loading phase, in order the filling of muscles to be successful.Between meals, posing is obligatory, so that carbohydrates can enter the muscles and form glycogen.Since insulin sensitivity is sky-high,its spike from pancreas may lead to lethargic state.Vanadium (Vanadyl Sulfate) and alpha lipoic acid (ALA) assist in this process as they act as they mimic insulin's action. Fast-acting insulin is the ideal solution, but it carries the risk of water retention in the subcutaneous and the cause of lipogenesis.

Therefore its use has to be accordingly to conditioning of the particular athlete.As known, carbohydrates have the ability to bind water and the formation of muscle glycogen.One molecule of carb requires four molecules of starch,in order glycogen to be synthesized. There sweet spot-borderline between muscle fullness and water retention under the skin, has to be found. This task depends highly under the experienced coach of each athlete.Onion skin look equals to neglible film of fluid kept under epidermis.

The last day before the show, water intake has to be minimized.

Usually athletes tend to restrict water during the last twelve hours before prejudging.During this time period, we can drink sips of cold water and suck ice cubes.A tricky method would be to measure the amount of fluid we diurate and drink half of it afterwards.This will ensure less water will be presented in the system.

Regular massage can be helpful,by increasing blood and lymphatic flow.This muscle relaxation can improve separation, the ability of muscles to show up.Legs during bedtime should be kept at 30 degrees inclined position. The reason is that this posture prevents swelling and edema coming from gravity.

Quite many athletes have one or more tattoos on various parts of their body. Even though I have enough (which I got them along the way), I do believe that the fewer and non-visible tattoos are, the better is.

Bodybuilding

Even from aesthetic point of view, but also from separation perspective.

The morning of the show, three hours at least before prejudging, we should have a breakfast rich in calories. Breakfast should contain a high sodium food, such as a burger, as long as we don't drink water at all.

Fat also plays a role, of satiety feeling, while it also provides sustained energy source, during the hard time between comparisons.Warming up at the back stage area has to be done in appropriate way.We don't need muscles to become blocky and sweaty.The less a body sweats, the drier it actually is.

Just before hitting on stage, a spoon of honey and red wine can help with vascularity.Honey and simple carbs bring high osmolality and make veins to swell, will alcohol ensured vasodilation.Supplements that can also assist on that are arginine,citrulline,yohimbine,niacin and glycerin.

Viagra overdose leads to extensive vasodilation, resulting in hot flushes, headaches and hypotension.Clenbuterol and ephedrine are strictly prohibited, because the can lead to dehydration and spasms, but also to peripheral vasoconstriction.The use of diuretics depends upon each individual.Usually advanced athletes use spironolactone (aldactone), which is a potassium sparring diuretic.Potassium is the main intracellular electrolyte, so muscles are still able to look full (volumised).However,spironolactone's abuse can lead to life threatening hyperkalemia and myocardial arrhythmia (ventricular fibrillation). The use of salbutamol inhaler can actually improve VO2max and breathing process. Stress leads to the production of cortisol (and aldosterone), that can actually ruin the physique.

In case body looks extremely dry just few minutes before hitting the stage, a bit of salt can make physique look even better; as long as water intake is out of the question. As known, sodium is the main extracellular element and fills up the intracellular space, leading to swelling and increased osmolality. This will eventually make muscles to look more pumped and jacked.

POSSING

Posing in the sport of bodybuilding is about isometric contractions, in which the length of the muscle remains unchanged.

Before we hit a pose, we take a deep breath and exhale gradually throughout the pose that lasts around five seconds. Posing requires excellent physical condition especially during the demanding comparison rounds.In a bodybuilding event is not your body that is being evaluated, but your physique as you represent it to the judges. Emphasizing your strong body parts, while hiding your weaknesses is the best possible way.

The sport of bodybuilding is basically an illusion and peak has to be achieved in proper timing.Not the day before, or the following day of the show.

The art of posing requires hours of preparation and evaluation by an experienced observer.Moreover it represents one of the four parameters assessed. The way you feel about yourself, reflects on stage and to the judges.Symmetry and balance, is among the key criteria for winning a competition. Mainly is a matter of pure genetic, but always can get improved through proper training.

By the term hardness in bodybuilding, we mean the granite look, depending on a variety of factors.

Firstly, it has to do with the low fat percentage.As known, subcutaneous tissue holds estrogens and estrogens equal to fluid retention.But it's also a matter of water retention under the skin, even though body fat percentage is close to five percent.These facts will make body to appear smooth and puffy.

Secondly, training with free heavy weights and lesser reps range can make the physique to look more dense, thick and solid.

Thirdly, the amount of androgens (and aromatase inhibitors presented, able to oxidize and minimize fat tissue (testosterone, drostenolone,fluoxymesterone, mesterolone & anastrozol, letrozole, exemestane).

The signs of an ultra ripped body (<6%) include:

Erector spinae muscle group (lower back), with the reveal of Christmas tree.

Also the crispy look of external obliques and serratus anterior muscles (gills).

Hamstrings separation is always a hard one to achieve (biceps femoris, semitendinosus, semimembranosus).

Without any doubt the gluteus maximus striations is the toughest among all.

It is the result of training,dieting,drug use and genetics as well.

The mandatory poses involve the front look, the side and the rear.

In this way there is a comprehensive assessment and evaluation of the overall appearance.

The front poses involve relax posing, that practically shows the "V"-taper and reverse triangular shape (tiny midsection,shoulder width).

The front double biceps and also the front lats spread.The abdominal-legs pose reveals quadriceps separation, along with rectus abdominis and external oblique muscles.

Finally the most muscular pose (or the crab pose), where trapezoids, arms and deltoids are revealed in all their glory.

Bodybuilding

On side poses we have the side chest pose and the side triceps pose.

At rear poses respectively we have the rear lats spread and rear double biceps. Keep in mind that an athlete can show a different look from the front to the rear, depending majorly in water and fat retention (buttocks, lower back and hams).

EPILOGUE

WHAT BODYBUILDING IS ALL ABOUT?

Bodybuilding is a highly demanding sport.Discipline diet, exhaustive exercise, sacrifices in personal matters, financial demands make the iron sport to be an extreme one.A physique requires decades of practice, in order to achieve perfection.Quality of muscle is accomplished with years of continuous practice.Bodybuilding does not only involve physical stamina and charisma.Mentality, positive thinking, courage, persistence are skills that play an essential role; especially during the hard time of precontest preparation.The champion should have the will and the skill; however the will, has to be stronger than the skill.

Bodybuilding is a subjective sport, where aesthetic criteria come into judgment.In other words, it is a sport of demonstration.Muscularity, definition, symmetry and posing are evaluated.

The iron sport has millions of fans worldwide, but quite many accusers as well.It's a highly contradictive sport, but very impressive too.Herculean physiques of modern champions will always inspire and be a motive for the youth.

Bodybuilding teaches you how to nourish your body in a healthy way.Teaches you to become a fighter, who never gives up and trains regularly with discipline.It's not just a matter of looks, but also of general physical condition, mind and body.It represents strength, stamina, endurance, health, beauty. It's a way of living and a lifestyle, not a casual sport, instead.Chemical enhancement and drug abuse is a matter of personal choice, according to everyone's goals and targets. But always remember that one day you will pay your dues and the price of your vanity.

A natural bodybuilding talent, with supreme genetics, should have the following characteristics:

1) abundance of white-fast twitch muscle fibers, rich in mitochondria,

2) wide clavicles-narrow midsection, along with small wrists

3) mesomorphic body type, with fast metabolic rate,

4) ambitious, aspiring, hard working, patient and methodical mind, with a persistent character.

Of course, someone who does not fulfill all these conditions does not mean he is a failure in bodybuilding. History has proved that with will and hard work and discipline, you can move on to some extent. In the sport of bodybuilding, the greatest factor comes to genetics. Delicate physiques are more aesthetic (Lee Labrada, Flex Wheeler, Dexter Jackson, Phil Heath, Bob Paris), while more solid structures appear to be more Herculean (Reg Park-RIP, Lou Ferrigno, Dorian Yates, Ronnie Coleman, Grec Kovacs-RIP, Nasser El Sonbaty-RIP). The talent is necessary to move on, but it's not enough on its own. Gifted, but lazy athletes have remained unchanged, although their great potential. Instead, aspiring and optimistic hard workers went much further ahead of their expectations. Discipline and deprivation took them to the top. It doesn't really matter how big the dog bites, but how hard he bites, instead.

The bodies of the 70s era, seemed more realistic and humane. They lacked freaky definition, ridiculous hardness, the impressive separation, the supreme muscularity. On the contrary, they were symmetrical, balanced, aesthetic, and proportional.Training was based on free weights workouts, sometimes even twice a day.The motto "mass with class" represented their philosophy.

No Frankenstein jaws, no protruding stomachs, no gorilla butts. Nothing but outstanding "V" taper shaped sculpted physiques.Nowadays, the iron sport is sort of a freak show, where mass is king and size does matter.After all, it's million dollar fitness industry. Spectators and audience are excited with mass monsters, when they hit the most muscular pose.Bodybuilding is a subjective sport, where Goliath does not always defeat David.Of course size matters, however bodybuilding has to do with the overall presence on stage, how beautifully developed a body as a whole is, as well as how to present it to the judges, the art of posing, and the overall appearance.As Arnold said: "it's not your physique that is being evaluated; it's your body as you represent it, into the judges after all".Although there are four main criteria (muscularity, definition, symmetry and posing), each judge may have different perspective to them.Therefore, there will always be deviations in results and athletes will fell they got "robbed".This is a classic phenomenon that occurs even from a local amateur contest, to the ultimate professional show, the Mr. Olympia.

Mind is the strongest muscle and it controls the body,as seven (1979-1975,1980) times Mr Olympia,Arnold Schwatzenegger said.You need a vision in order to stay hungry and accomplish your goals.When is a want,there is a will and a way.Nothing is impossible and dreams come true,if you believe in them.

Bodybuilding

If I were "Dr. Frankenstein", I would create the "ideal" body consisting of different body parts, taken from the following athletes:

1) CHEST: Arnold Schwarzenegger & Lee Haney,

2) BACK: Dorian Yates & Ronnie Coleman,

3) DELTS: Kevin Levrone & Kenneth '"Flex" Wheeler,

4) TRAPS: Marcus Ruhl & Nasser El Sonbaty,

5) QUADS: Tom Plats & Paul De Mayo,

6) HAMS: Branch Warren & Tom Prince,

7) GLUTES: Richy Gaspari & Kai Greene,

8) CALVES: Mike Matarazo & Jay Cutler,

9) BICEPS: Robbie Robinson & Philip Heath,

10) TRICEPS: Andreas Muntzer & Ernie Taylor,

11) FOREARMS: Sergio Oliva & Lee Priest,

12) ABS: Shawn Ray & Dexter Jackson.

George Touliatos

BODYBUILDING AND MORTALITY

Several professionals of which the competitions I grew up with passed away the last couple of years, most of betrayed by their hearts.

Doping abuse requires some time, in order to establish irreversible health consequences.

Famous IFBB pro's who died, include the following:

1) Matt Duval (USA)

2) Art Artwood (CAN)

3) Ed Van Amsterdam (HOL)

4) Nasser El Sonbaty (EGY)

5) Greg Kovac (CAN)

6) Mike Matarazzo (USA)

7) Daniele Seccarecci (ITA)

8) Baito Abbaspour (IRN)

9) Dallas Mc Carver (USA)

10) Rich Piana (USA)

Also, the Americans Don Long and Tom Prince, suffered acute renal failure and had to undergo kidney dialysis, for life. One of the greatest talents, the promising American Dennis Newman developed leukemia-fortunately healed, shortly after winning his IFBB Pro card in 1994 (NPC overall winner). We shouldn't neglect the very first victim, Arab Mohammed Benaziza (Momo-Giand Killer). He tragically died of diuretics abuse (spironolactone) and severe dehydration at the Dutch grand prix in 1993. Potassium sparing diuretics lead to electrolyte ibalances,known as jyperkalemia. This can lead to fatal heart arrhythmia,suck as ventricular tachycardia.

Three years later, the Austrian Andreas Muntzer at age of 31 in 1996.It was just three weeks after his last participation in Arnold Schwarzenegger Classic. He was admitted to hospital with intense stomach pains. During surgery an extensive hepatic tumor was revealed, along with undissolved pills were found in his stomach. An autopsy revealed atrophic adrenals, atrophic testicles and heart enlargement, twice as much the normal weight. Muntzer was speculated to have abused a cortisol blocker (aminoglutethimide), leading to severe secondary Addison's disease and insufficiency. His cardiomegaly was the result of somatropin abuse, while his testicular atrophy was a common side effect of steroid abuse, without the use of HCG.

Of course there are other professionals who died later in life, such as the legendary Mike Mentzer betrayed by his heart in 2001 at his 50th birthday.Moreover, the mythical Sergio Oliva (1967-1968-1969 Mr.Olympia) and legendary Serge Nubre the same age, of 70 years.Nubre was hospitalised for almost a month, until he passed away in coma.

Mr. Universe and Mr. America and actor Steve Reeves from Non-Hodgkin Lymphoma in 2000 at 74. The iconic South African, Reg Park from malignant melanoma in 2007, at 79 years old.

In the summer of 2017,two young famous professionals died. Rich Piana from cardiovascular issues at 46 and Dallas Mc Garver (ASC USA first runner up) so young at 26 from same issues.

Last but not least, the first Mr. Olympia in history (1965-1966 Mr.Olympia), Larry Scott at the age of 75.

Lately the sultan of symmetry,four times ASC winner and two times Mr.Olympia runner up Keneth Flex Wheeler was partially amputated in his right leg. Rumors speculate it was linked to poor circulation as a result of his kidney transplant,or perhaps vasculopathy coming from DM2 and GH abuse.

While most recently two times Mr.Olympia (1976,1981),Franko Columbu passed away from heart attack at the age of 78 in 2019.

It is an indisputable fact, that competitive bodybuilding deals with a minority of few genetically gifted (physically and mentally) individuals. However, for every dream in life, there is a price to pay for.

Unfortunately, quite many are willing to sacrifice their lives, even for the sake of their vanity and glory. Options that for others seem shallow and careless, especially for those who live with disabilities or chronic diseases. It seems unfair to be born with an organic failure. But it seems quite idiotic, end up with organic failure, as a result of your poor choices. Nature is smarter than people think; if you don't show respect to your health, you will regret it somehow someday.

TOP 100 BODYBUILDERS OF ALL TIME

-STEVE REEVES (RIP)
-REG PARK (RIP)
-VINCE GIRONDA (RIP)
-JOE GOLD (RIP)
-JOHN GRIMEK (RIP)
-ED CORNEY (RIP)
-BILL PEARL
-BOYER COE
-TONY PEARSON
-LARRY SCOT (RIP)
-SERGIO OLIVA (RIP)
-ARNOLD SCWARZENEGGER
-DAVE DRAPER
-FRANK ZANE
-LOU FERIGNO
-SERGE NUBRE (RIP)
-ROBBY ROBINSON
-ALBERT BECKLES
-DENNIS TINERINO (RIP)
-DANNY PADILA
-CASEY VIATOR (RIP)
-FRANCO COLUMBO (RIP)

-JUSUP WILKOSZ (RIP)
-MIKE MENTZER (RIP)
-TOM PLATS
-ALBERT BECKLES
-CHRIS DICKERSON
-SAMIR BANNOUT
-BERTIL FOX
-LEE HANEY
-MOHAMED MAKAWI
-BOB PARIS
-MIKE CHRISTIAN
-MIKE QUEEN
-RICHY GASPARI
-LEE LABRADA
-GARY STRYDOM
-BERRY DE MEY
-FRANCIS BENFATO
-RALPH MULLER
-PAVOL JABLONICKI
-GREG KOVAKS (RIP)
-GRAIG TITUS
-SONNY SCHMIDT (RIP)
-EDDIE ROBBINSON
-EDUARDO KAWAK (RIP)

Bodybuilding

- PAUL DE MAYO (RIP)
- SHAWN RAY
- MOHAMED BENAZIZA (RIP)
- CHARLES CLAIRMONT
- DARREM CHARLES
- DORIAN YATES
- ANDREAS MUNTZER (RIP)
- KEVIN LEVRONE
- PACO BAUTISTA
- ED VAN AMSTERDAM (RIP)
- PAUL DILLET
- MELVIN ANTONY
- MIKE FRANCOIS
- ERNIE TAYLOR
- VINCE TAYLOR
- NASSER EL SONBATY (RIP)
- JEAN PIER FUX
- BOB CHICHERILO
- ART ARTWOOD (RIP)
- GUNTER SCHLIERKAMP
- RONNIE COLEMAN
- KENNETH "FLEX" WHEELER
- DEXTER JACKSON
- JOHNNIE JACKSON

-JAY CUTLER
-MILOS SARCEV
-GEORGE FARAH
-KING KAMALI
-AHMAD HAIDAR
-MARCUS RUHL
-MIKE MATARAZO (RIP)
-CHRIS CORMIER
-LEE PRIEST
-TROY ALVES
-GUSTAVO BADEL
-HIDEDATA YAMAGISHI
-DENNIS JAMES
-DENNIS WOLF
-RONIE ROCKEL
-VICTOR MARTINEZ
-TONEY FREEMAN
-PHIL HEATH
-KAI GREEN
-BRANCH WARREN
-FLEX LEWIS
-DALLAS MC GARVER (RIP)
-EVAN CENTOPANI

Bodybuilding

-HADI CHOOPAN
-BEN PAKULSKI
-BAITO ABBASPOUR (RIP)
-MAMDOUH ELSSBIAY
-CEDRIC MC MILLAN
-SHAWN RHODEN
- BRANDON CURRY

SELF CRITISISM

If have regretted the use of chemical enhancement, it is mainly due to two reasons (as I have mentioned in one of my interviews):

1) Because of my health issues (LV hypertrophy, intramuscular abscess-hospitalised,heart arrythmias-hospitalised, dehydration-hospitalised,pharmaceutical hepatitis, atheromatosis-statins administration, roid rage-psychotherapy, hypogonadism-TRT).

2) Because AAS & PED's abuse costed me in terms of social relationships with relatives-family, friends-colleagues, relationships-marriage (divorce).

I had to isolate from people and society in general, in order to improve my physique, while I was spending all of my savings for my preparation: drugs, supplements, food, massage, tanning.

I almost felt just like a junkie, who was desperately searching for his dope in order to feel better, or perform better at the gym, or even to improve his sexual performance.I became occasionally psychotic (misconceptions), as a result of highly androgenic compounds (halotestin-trenbolone) and bipolar (manic-depressive) under the psychological effect of CNS stimulants (ephedrine-clenbuterol).

My roid rage was so severe, that forced me into violence against materials, objects and mostly got me into fights.But mostly, I am sorry I let down my parents and my ex wife.Since shows and PCT were through, several times I faced severe depression, while life seemed empty, unreal, and meaningless.Mood swings and emotional instability were quite common symptoms.Since bodybuilding was not my main priority, it was hard to accept that the party was over, while I had to focus on my medical practice and biopathology in particular.I had to give a valiant struggle with my inner demons and push it to the limit; basically it was equal of a rehabilitation process that I went through.

I wish I knew back then, what I know now; I thought I was a kind of a superman and someone special with supreme looks.But I was just another egopath, selfish, arrogant, who tried to earn self respect from his vanity.Definitely I was suffering from Adonis complex and muscle dysmorphia (reverse anorexia nervosa).I was totally obsessed with my body image and the way people looked at me.

Competitive bodybuilders are potentially insecure individuals with a sick body and an ill mind.And by that, what I mean is that "whatever shines, ain't gold".It is the other side of the coin, the one that is rarely revealed and usually people tend to hide- or avoid it, simply cause truth hurts.

This is a sincere confession of a former competitive bodybuilder, who sacrificed several aspects of his life, in order to accomplish one of his life time dreams.All of my wisdom and knowledge is enclosed within my books.I did it in order to protect the others and make them to avoid my mistakes.At least choose for their decisions, knowing the price they have to pay for their vain goals.

It seems unfair to be born with one kidney, but it seems idiotic ending up with one kidney, as a result of your poor choices.Knowledge is power, while ignorance is dangerous. Nature is smarter than people think and one day you might pay the price of your vanity.Knowledge is power,while ignorance is dangerous and illusion of knowledge even worse.

REFERENCES

WILLIAM LLEWWELLIN - ANABOLICS 11th edition 2017

MICHAEL SCALLY, M.D. - Anabolic Steroids - A Question of Muscle: Human Subject Abuses in Anabolic Steroid Research, First edition (December 31, 2008)

JAY CAMBELL- The Definitive Testosterone Replacement Therapy Manual, 2015

JOHN CRISLER DR - Testosterone Replacement Therapy: A Recipe for Success, 2015

NELSON VERGEL- Testosterone: A Man's Guide- 2nd edition 2011

MASSIMO SPATTINI-ANTIAGING, 2016

WWW.PATRICARNOLDBLOG.COM

Marshall B. Dunning BS, MS, PhD, Frances Fischbach RN- Manual of Laboratory and Diagnostic Tests, 9th edition 2014

Murray, R. Et al. Harpers Illustrated Biochemistry. McGraw Hill Education; 30th edition 2015

Koeppen, B. Stanton, B. Berne & Levy Physiology. Mosby; 6th edition 2010

Harrison's Principles of Internal Medicine, 19th edition 2016

GARY WADLER, Brian Hainline, M.D. - DRUGS AND THE ATHLETE, April 1989

David R. Mottram, Neil Chester- DRUGS IN SPORTS, 6th edition 2014

DAN DUCHAINE - UNDERGROUND STEROID HANDBOOK, 1988

JULIUS A.VIDA-ANDROGENS AND ANABOLIC AGENTS: Chemistry And Pharmacology

STAVROS CHATZOS-DOPING, A PUBLIC HEALTH ISSUE, 2004

THOMAS O'CONNOR-AMERICA ON STEROIDS,A TIME TO HEAL 2017

Chitturi S, Farrell GC. Adverse effects of hormones and hormone antagonists on the liver. In, Kaplowitz N, DeLeve LD, eds. Drug-induced liver disease. 3rd ed. Amsterdam: Elsevier, 2013, pp. 605-20. (Review of hepatotoxicity of androgenic steroids including cholestasis, vascular disorders, benign tumors and hepatocellular carcinoma).

Mumoli N, Cei M, Cosimi A. "Drug-related hepatotoxicity". N. Engl. J. Med. 2006; 354 (20): 2191–3

Philipp Solbach, Andrej Potthoff, et al. Testosterone-receptor positive hepatocellular carcinoma in a 29-year old bodybuilder with a history of anabolic androgenic steroid abuse: a case report BMC Gastroenterol. 2015; 15: 60

Ursodeoxycholic acid and bile-acid mimetics as therapeutic agents for cholestatic liver diseases: an overview of their mechanisms of action. Poupon R. Clin Res Hepatol Gastroenterol. 2012 Sep; 36 Suppl 1:S3-12. doi: 10.1016/S2210-7401(12)70015-3

Peter J Angell, Neil Chester, et al. Performance enhancing drug abuse and cardiovascular risk in athletes: implications for the clinician. Br J Sports Med 2012; 46: i78-i84

Manu Kaushik, Siva P. Sontineni, et al. Cardiovascular disease and androgens: A review. International Journal of Cardiology 2010; 142: 8–14

H Kuipers, et al. Prospective echocardiographic assessment of androgenic-anabolic steroids effects on cardiac structure and function in strength athletes.Int J Sports Med 2003; 24: 344-351

Ma F, Liu D. 17β-trenbolone, an anabolic-androgenic steroid as well as an environmental hormone, contributes to neurodegeneration. Toxicol Appl Pharmacol. 2015, 1; 282(1):68-76

Francesco P. Busardò, Paola Frati et al. The Impact of Nandrolone Decanoate on the Central Nervous System. Curr Neuropharmacol. 2015, 13(1): 122–131

O'Connor DB, Archer J, Wu FC. Effects of testosterone on mood, aggression, and sexual behavior in young men: a double-blind, placebo-controlled, cross-over study. J Clin Endocrinol Metab. 2004, 89(6):2837-45

Cristoforo Pomara, Margherita Neri et al. Neurotoxicity by Synthetic Androgen Steroids: Oxidative Stress, Apoptosis, and Neuropathology: A Review. Curr Neuropharmacol. 2015 ; 13(1): 132–145

Leal C. Herlitz, Glen S. Markowitz, et al. Development of Focal Segmental Glomerulosclerosis after Anabolic Steroid Abuse. J Am Soc Nephrol. 2010; 21(1): 163–172

Safa E. Almukhtar, Alaa A. Abbas, et al. Acute kidney injury associated with androgenic steroids and nutritional supplements in bodybuilders. Clinical Kidney Journal, 2015; 8 (4): 415–419

Patrick Harrington, Galil Ali, et al. The development of focal segmental glomerulosclerosissecondary to anabolic steroid abuse. BMJ Case Reports 2011; doi:10.1136/bcr.07.2011.4531

Pendergraft WF, Herlitz LC, et al. Nephrotoxic effects of common and emerging drugs. Clin J Am Soc Nephrol 2014; (9): 1996–2005

Amit Momaya, Marc Fawal, Reed Este. Performance-Enhancing Substances in Sports: A Review of the Literature. Sports Medicine 2015; 45, (4): 517-531

Kenneth P. Barnes, Catherine R. Rainbow. Update on Banned Substances 2013. Sports Health. 2013; 5, (5): 442-447

Werner W. Franke, Brigitte Berendonk. Hormonal doping and androgenization of athletes: a secret program of the German Democratic Republic government. Clinical Chemistry 1997; 43, (7): 1262-1279

C Dufour, J Svahn, et al. Front-line immunosuppressive treatment of acquired aplastic anemia. Bone Marrow Transplantation 2013; (48): 174-177

Jenny Erkander Mullen, et al. Perturbation of the Hematopoietic Profile by Anabolic Androgenic Steroids. Journal of Hormones 2014;

M. Maggio, P. J. Snyder, G. P. Ceda et al. Is the haematopoietic effect of testosterone mediated by erythropoietin? The results of a clinical trial in older men, Andrology 2013; (1): 24-28

S. Shahani, M. Braga-Basaria, et al. Androgens and erythropoiesis: past and present. Journal of Endocrinological Investigation 2009; (32):704-716

Papanayiotou P, Marketos S. Renal effects of a new anabolic steroid (29'038-Ba) in old age. Pharmacol.Clin. 1968; (2):43-6

Amin Z1, Canli T, Epperson CN. Effect of estrogen-serotonin interactions on mood and cognition. Behav Cogn Neurosci Rev. 2005 Mar;4(1):43-58

Dawson-Hughes B, Stern D, Goldman J, Reichlin S. Regulation of growth hormone and somatomedin-C secretion in postmenopausal women: effect of physiological estrogen replacement.J Clin Endocrinol Metab. 1986 Aug;63(2):424-32

Hartgens F, Kuipers H Effects of androgenic-anabolic steroids in athletes. Sports Med. 2004; 34 (8):513-54

Achar S, Rostamian A, Narayan SM. Cardiac and metabolic effects of anabolic-androgenic steroid abuse on lipids, blood pressure, left ventricular dimensions, and rhythm. Am J Cardiol. 2010 Sep 15; 106 (6): 893-901

Hengevoss J, et al. Combined effects of androgen anabolic steroids and physical activity on the hypothalamic-pituitary-gonadal axis. J Steroid Biochem Mol Biol.2015 Jun; 150:86-96

Farzad Gheshlaghi, et al. Cardiovascular manifestations of anabolic steroids in association with demographic variables in body building athletes. J Res Med Sci. 2015 Feb; 20 (2): 165–168.

Peter J Angell, Neil Chester, et al. Performance enhancing drug abuse and cardiovascular risk in athletes: implications for the clinician. Br J Sports Med 2012; 46: i78-i84

Manu Kaushik, Siva P. Sontineni, et al. Cardiovascular disease and androgens: A review. International Journal of Cardiology 2010; 142: 8–14

Dawson-Hughes B, Stern D, Goldman J, Reichlin S. Regulation of growth hormone and somatomedin-C secretion in postmenopausal women: effect of physiological estrogen replacement. J Clin Endocrinol Metab. 1986 Aug;63(2):424-32

Finkelstein, Joel. Et al. Gonadal Steroids and Body Composition, Strength, and Sexual Function. The New England Journal of Medicine. Sept 2013

Holt RI, Sönksen PH. Growth hormone, IGF-I and insulin and their abuse in sport. Br J Pharmacol. 2008 Jun; 154(3):542-56

INTERVIEW

About The Author: George Touliatos

Interview by Tim Zakowski on January 31st, 2016

for anabolic.org

Thank you for taking the time to do this interview George, many of our readers are very curious to learn more about you. After all, it isn't every day that people see a doctor from Greece, with the physique of a pro bodybuilder, who is known the world over for his knowledge of anabolic steroids. How did your passion for performance enhancing drugs develop, and at what age?

George Touliatos: First of all, I want to thank you for giving me the opportunity to do this interview. While I never became a pro bodybuilder, I was a competitive amateur bodybuilder who managed to win twice at the nationals. I am very glad to be a member of the Anabolic.org family and I feel most thankful to William Llewellyn, the author of ANABOLICS, and founder of Molecular Nutrition, Anabolic.org and ROIDTEST. I was a huge fan of his work from the time I was doing my residency in biopathology. My first mentor actually suggested that I study William's ANABOLICS book, almost ten years ago. Honestly, I had never thought of what life holds in store; that almost a decade later I would have the privilege of being his associate.

Therefore, I feel blessed being able to accomplish this dream of a lifetime, as athletic performance was my passion since my early years.

We are just as happy to have you as part of the family George. Did your interest in learning about steroids lead you into studying medicine, and ultimately into your career as a doctor? While studying, what was the one subject that fascinated you the most?

GT: Among my dreams as a teenager, was to become a professional athlete, or a physical education teacher. However, the fact that I came from a conservative medical family influenced me towards sports medicine science and functional anatomy. This was my favourite subject during my academic years in medicine. There was a direct correlation between myology, meaning skeletal muscles nomenclature and bodybuilding training. Therefore, I was able to understand how a particular exercise works, by knowing the origin-insertion of the muscle belly. Athletics were a top priority of mine early on, and weight lifting/bodybuilding later became my focus during my academic years as a medical student. I was good mainly in sprinting and the long jump early in my life. This is something common among guys who later start resistance training, because it involves the same kind of (fast-twitch) muscle fibers. I took part in several events and managed to win several medals between 1982-1991 at Athens College.

Later, during my Pre-Medical course in Budapest (1991, Semmelweiss University), I joined the gym and soon realized that I had the ability to gain size quite easily. I believe my body type was meso-endomorphic. At that time, I had no idea about nutrition basics, or even supplementation. I was 18 years old and weighed around 170 pounds, at 5ft 9 inches tall. Supplementation came later, in 1997 I tried the basic stuff such as protein powders (back then the milk and egg combination was still popular), amino acids, vitamins, EFAs, HMB and creatine monohydrate. I do remember that

supplementation was more expensive back then, compared to today. Mind that, specialized nitric oxide formulas were not yet available. However, thermogenic supplementation was still on the market and legal. They were far more effective than current formulas, due to the inclusion of mahuang-ephedra herbs.

Soon after I graduated from Athens Medical School, in the summer of 1999, I moved to Kefalonia Island (West Greece, IonianSea) in order to work as a General Practitioner. That period literally changed my life for the better; it was the moment when I entered into the magical world of chemical enhancement and Performance Enhancing Drugs. Among my closest friends was a steroid guru, Simon, who noticed my natural talent and good symmetry and aesthetic physique. We shared the same passion, so we started training together, talking for hours about bodybuilding, training, nutrition and steroids. We even exchanged the FLEX & MuscleMag magazines, trying to learn as much as we could. Notice that there was no internet available back then and the only source was Dan Duchaine's handbook, a pioneer for that time. Being honest, during the early years I had no basic knowledge about AAS, but the fact I was a post graduate of Med school gave me the ability to understand physiology and endocrinology better. I had the privilege to perform blood work quite often at the public hospitals and understand the fluctuations of my biochemical and hormonal labs. This gave me an advantage to realize how drugs work and how supplementation, dieting and training affect the bodily systems. It was a valuable experience without any doubt, that I later introduced into the books that I wrote from 2012-2016.

Basically, the drugs came into my life after I became a doctor in 1999. I had the opportunity to judge better, being able to understand the significance of medical prevention rules. Of course, this may sound contradictory to some, however sometimes you do not think-or act as a scientist. You are driven from your passion and you turn on your other (athletic) side. There is a major difference between individuals who use PED's for cosmetic purposes, driven from vanity, and those who use them to become more competitive in sports, with a massive desire to win. The main reason I started abusing AAS &PED's was in order to enter into competitions. My first bodybuilding show took place at the age of 26, while I was still practicing as a General Practitioner. When people used to ask me, how the heck I was using chemical enhancement even though I was an MD, I mentioned the poor living habits of other colleagues (tobacco, alcohol, junk food, cocaine, lack of physical activity). Plus, there is the fact that AAS/PED's were medically prescribed for the treatment of certain diseases, including anemia, osteopenia, hypogonadism, and muscle wasting. Of course, back then I felt powerful and not vulnerable at all. Perhaps it was part of my arrogance, lack of experience and ignorance.

Describe the availability of anabolic steroids in Greece. Here in the USA, for example, nearly all of the supply is underground steroids with questionable validity. Are there true pharmaceutical grade options in Greece?

GT: AAS &PED's in Greece are available in pharmacy stores, and the majority of them do not require a medical prescription paper from a physician. The law is quite loose here and the only issue you face with underground marketing (non pharmaceutical compounds) is the penalty of financial crime. I know that law in USA-CAN-AUS is very strict and AAS-PED's legally resemble the class three of narcotics in Greece, (for instance diazepam, codeine). This is the list of drugs available at my local drug stores:

Bodybuilding

1) Testosterone Enanthate 250mg (Norma Hellas),

2) Testim gel (Ferring),

3) Decadurabolin 50mg (Organon),

4) Proviron tabs 25mg (Schering-Bayern),

5) Restadol caps 40mg (Organon),

6) Nolvadex tabs 10/20mg (AstraZeneca),

7) Pregnyl 1500/5000 iu (Organon),

8) Clomiphene citrate 50mg (Anfarm),

9) Spiropent 5mg/5ml (Boehringer Ingelheim),

10) Arimidex 1mg (AstraZeneca),

11) Femara 2.5mg (Novartis),

12) Aromasin 25mg (Pfizer),

13) Humulin N (Lilly),

14) Genotropin 16iu (Pfizer),

15) T3/T4 25mg (Unipharma),

16) Reductil 15mg (Abbott).

Prescription parer is needed for: Nandrolone, Somatropin and Amphetamines. All the rest are available without a prescription. Mind that before 2000, there was also the availability of Flouoxymesterone (Halotestin), Methenolone (Primobolan Depot) and even before Oxymetholone (Anasterone), stanozolol (Winstrol).

Wow, that is remarkable. Back to your days of competitive bodybuilding, what are some of your most exciting memories of competing?

GT: Concerning competitive bodybuilding, I have performed 12 shows.

I started in 2000 (age 26, at 175lbs) and competed until the masters in 2013 (age 40, at 200lbs). I won in 2000 (fitness class) and in 2009 (light heavyweight class). I remember the first time I won, at age 27, when I took the microphone in order to thank few people who had helped me. And I could not neglect of course, the moment when I doubled my victories nine years later. That was quite an achievement, trying my best for a comebackand knowing that I had to face guys ten years younger than me. It was very moving hearing my name as the winner. I have always been outspoken about my steroid abuse in the past. This was not for gossip, but in order to lighten up guys who lived in the shadows of ignorance, based on bro science. I spoke the truth with honesty and without hesitation, whether on live television, recorded appearances, radio shows, or in magazine and online interviews.

That is very noble of you George. On that note, what harm reduction tips would you like to share with our readers, in order to help protect their health and longevity while using AAS?

GT: As a medical doctor in Biopathology and a former steroid user, I have to provide information based on medical prevention rules. Proper lifestyle habits (no smoking, no narcotics, limited alcohol consumption, limited junk food, plenty of regular aerobic exercise, enough sleep every night) along with healthy nutrition and supplementation choices will ensure longevity. I recommend plenty of white meat, fish, vegetables, fruits, seeds and fiber. I recommend the avoidance of table salt and sugar, fried food, processed red meat, refined carbohydrates, trans and saturated fats, carbonated beverages, and gluten. These are among the basic rules that a health conscious steroid user should follow.

Additionally, you will want to perform regular lab work, regularly undergo a stress test/electrocardiogram to check the condition of your heart, and monitor your blood pressure regularly. If you're using methylated steroid tablets I recommend them to be taken sublingually, if using injectables be sure to rotate injection sites frequently. The use of supplements that support cardiovascular health and liver function, such as Molecular Nutrition Lipid and Liver Stabil is also advised. Be extra cautious with CNS stimulants, insulin and diuretics, as they are able to kill instantly in the case of overdose. Knowledge is power, while ignorance is dangerous. This is the motto that I have introduced within my books for the last four years.

And now for the final question and the one many readers will want to know the most: What was your favourite cycle that you ever ran? I'm curious about the compounds, dosages and duration.

GT: I have tried almost every injectable and several orals. The only noteworthy oral drugs I didn't have the chance to try were M3 (methyltrienolone) and THG (tetrahydrogestrinone). My highest abuse during pre-contest preparation was: During the last two weeks before my final show (2013 masters>40), I took the following PED's on a daily basis: 50mg fluoxymesterone, 50mg oxandrolone, 50mg stanozolol, 50mg exemestan (am/pm), 100mg mesterolone, 100mg testosterone suspension, 100mg trenbolone base, along with clenbuterol HCL, T3 and T4.

On the other hand, during the off season period of 2012, for a duration four weeks my peak on a weekly basis was: 2000mg testosterone enanthate, 1000mg nandrolone decaonate, 1000mg methenolone enanthate, 400mg parabolan, 50mg methandrostenolone ED, 100mg mesterolone and 40mg tamoxifen.

Thank you George, it was pleasure learning more about one of the brightest minds at Anabolic.org. You provide an incredible level of insight, being able to draw both from your

medical knowledge and first hand use. I, like the rest of our readers, will be looking forward to reading more articles from you in the near future!

GT: It was my pleasure giving you that exclusive interview. I am looking forward to publishing my latest book in the US market later this year. American readers are the world's experts and probably the most educated in this field. I have exchanged valuable information so far while working on it, and actually feel blessed being able to interact with some masterminds. Sincerely, GNT-MD

CV

George Touliatos is a physician, specialized in biopathology (2014)

He was a competitive bodybuilder and national light heavy weight champion (2000, 2009, 2010, 2013).

He is an expert on medical prevention and harm reduction regarding PEDsuse in sports and HRT in men.

He is a medical associate of Anabolics 11th edition (2017).

He is a medical contributor of the American Muscular Development magazine (2019) and online English, Spanish editions

He has his own weekly show on MD TV,

Ask Dr.Testosterone (2019)

He has extensively developed articles on Anabolic.org

(2015-2016)

He became a writer for steroidabuse.com (2019)

He is medical director for Balancemyhormones.co.uk (2019)

He has being a columnist for Greek editions of Musclemag & Muscular Development magazines (2014-2016)

George Touliatos was a medical associate for MYprotein.gr (2016-2017).

He was medical associate of Orthobiotiki.gr and Medihall.gr age management-preventive clinics in Athens, Greece

(2016-2019)

He has being tutor of ALS academy of Cyprus and peakperformance.gr academy in Greece (2015-2019)

He is author of four Greek books and three English in bodybuilding (2012, 2013, 2015,2017, 2018,2020)

He participated in several seminars across Greece and Cyprus, numerous TV and radio appearances, interviews in newspapers and websites between 2012-2019.

He entered medical congresses and festivals,regarding sports medicine and antiageing (2017-2019)

He was hosted five times by Super Human Radio of Kentucky (2015-2019), three by Muscular DevelopmentTV (2018), and RXMUSCLE (2018,2019), twice by TRTrevolution.com

(2016-2018) and once by Jay Cutler TV (2018). Also hosted by the Arnold Sports Festifal In Columbus OH (2020).

His personal website is gtoul.com (2014)

PICTURES

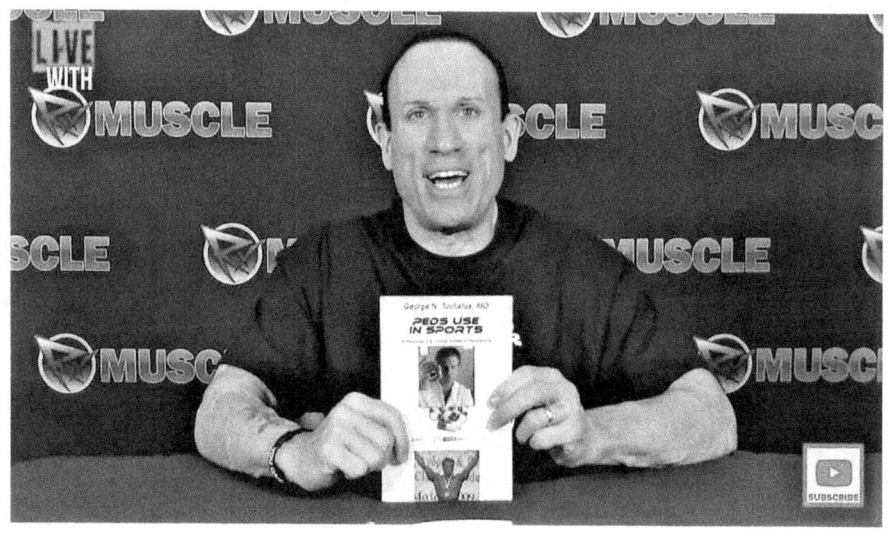

Dave Palumbo (USA)
NPC superheavy weights first runner up
Anabolic Freak columnist Muscular Development magazine
RXMUSCLE creator, Owner of Species Nutrition

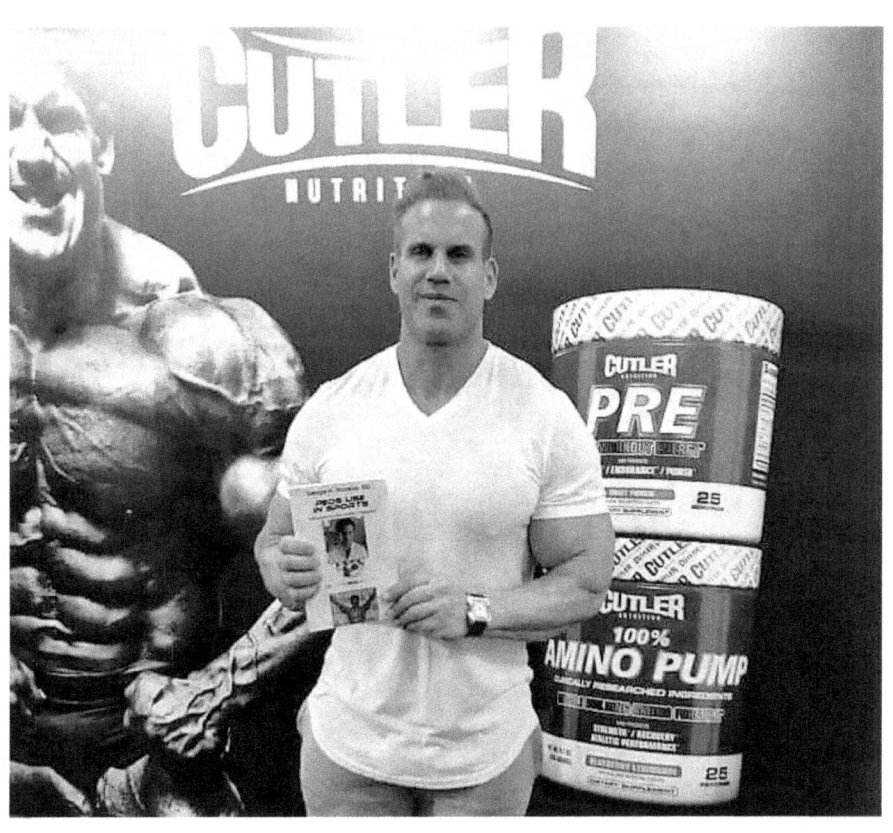

Jay Cutler (USA) Mr.Olympia 2006,2007,2009,2010
ASC USA 2002,2003,2004 champion
Owner of Cutler Nutrition

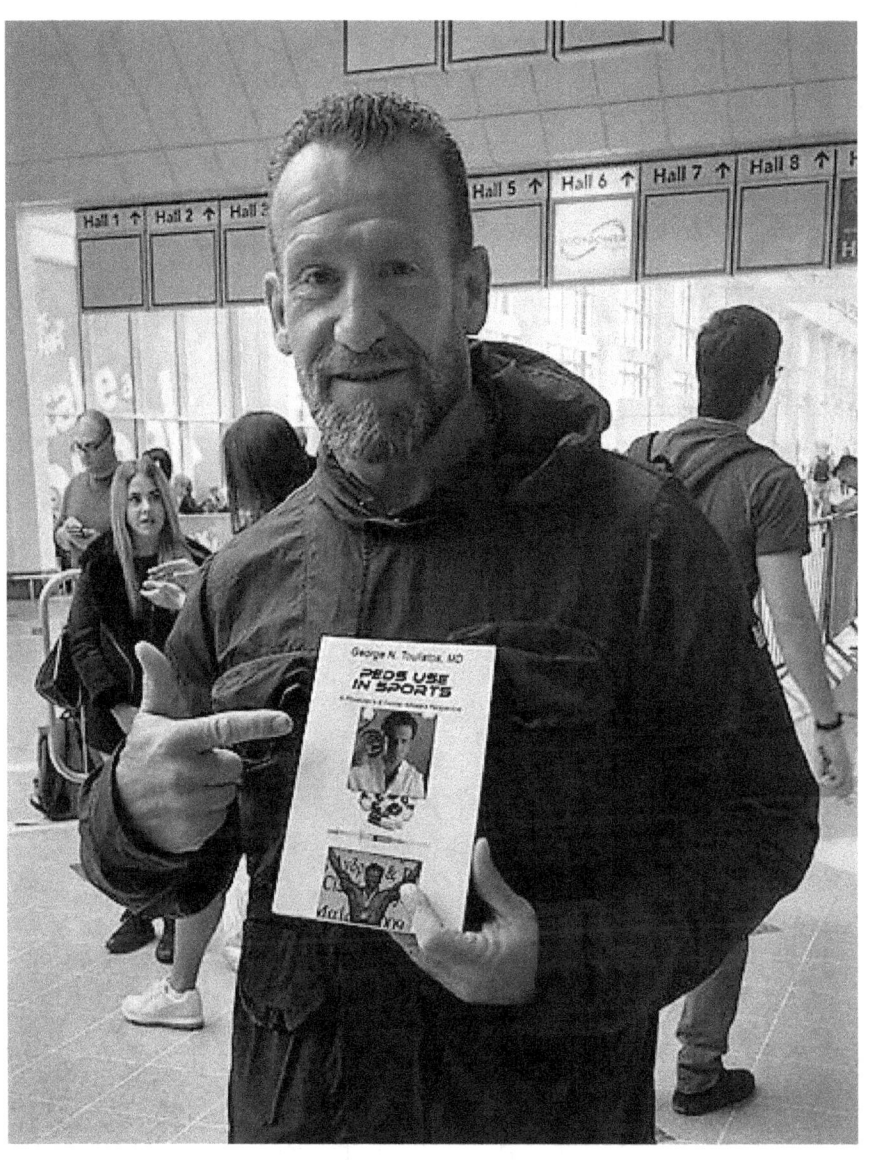

Dorian Yates (ENGLAND) Mr.Olympia 1992-1997
Owner of DY nutrition

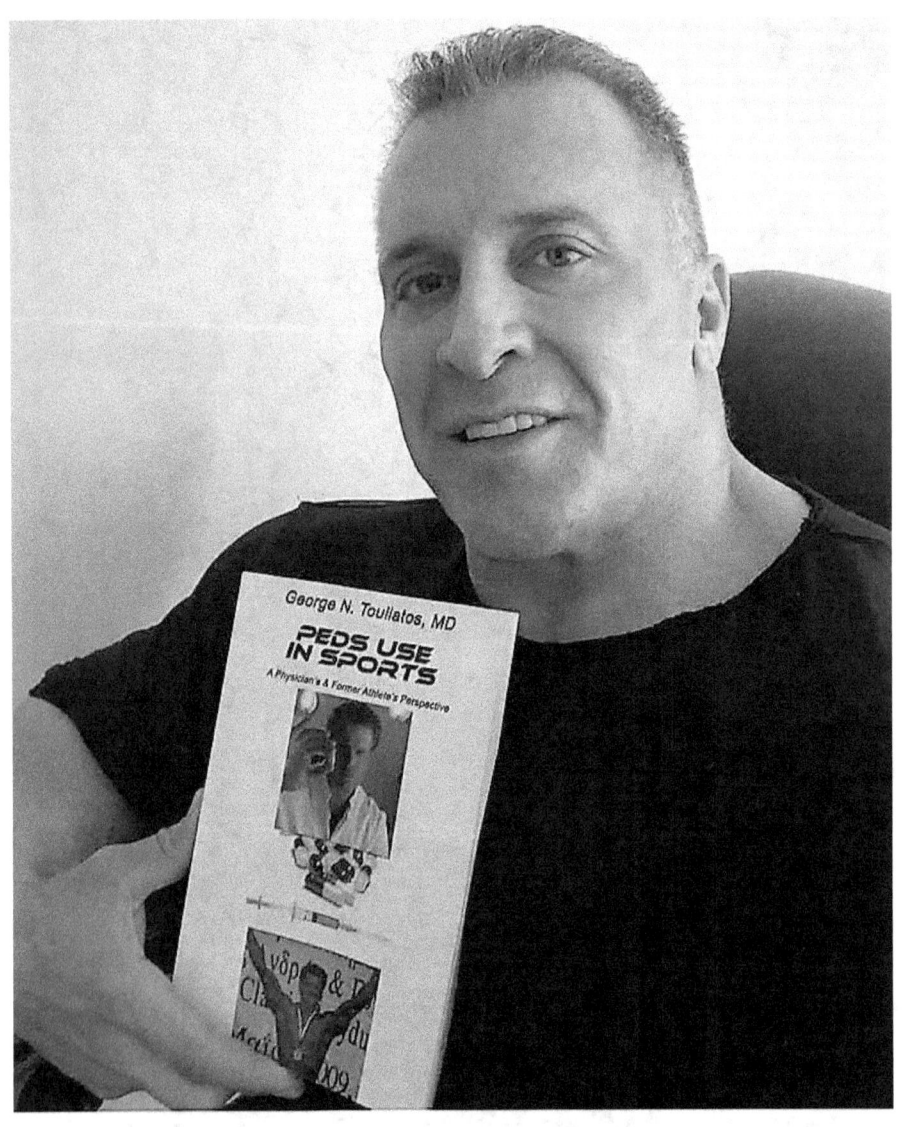

Milos Sarcev (SERBIA)

1997 Toronto Pro winner & Canada Pro winner

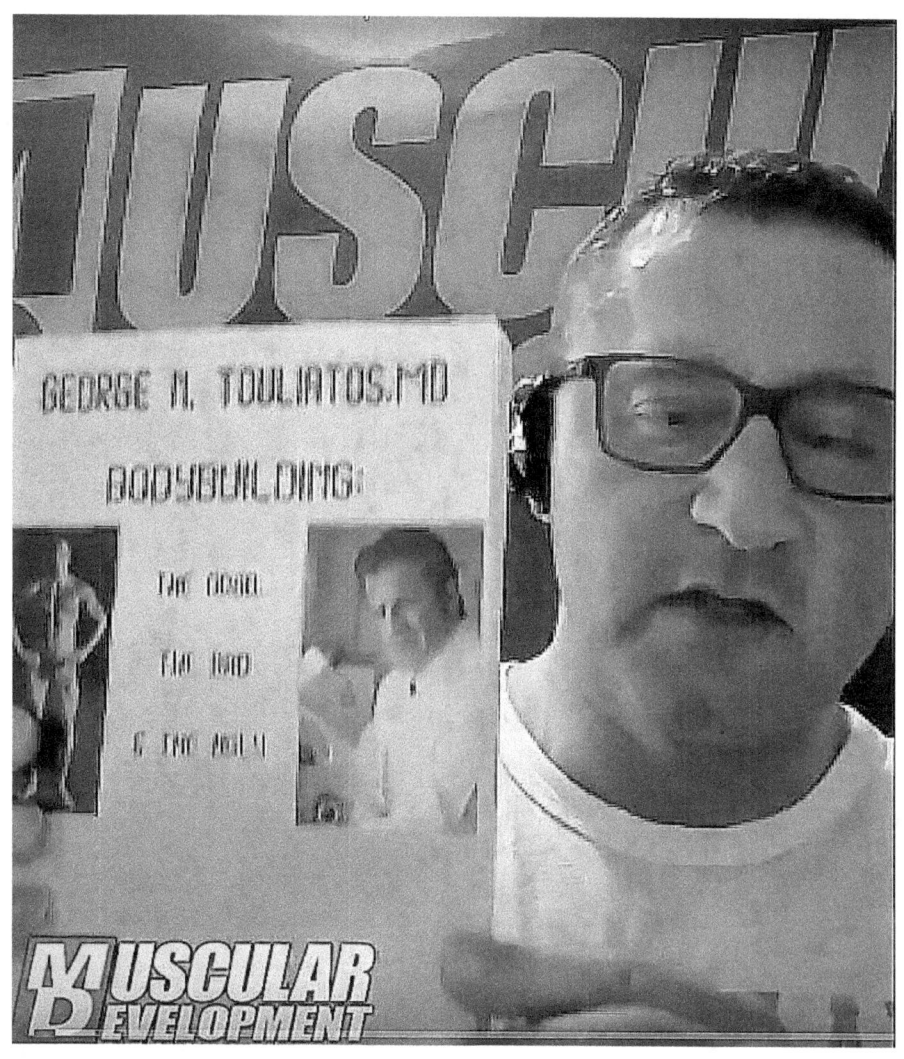

Ron Harris, Muscular Development online editor, bodybuilding writer, competitive bodybuilder.

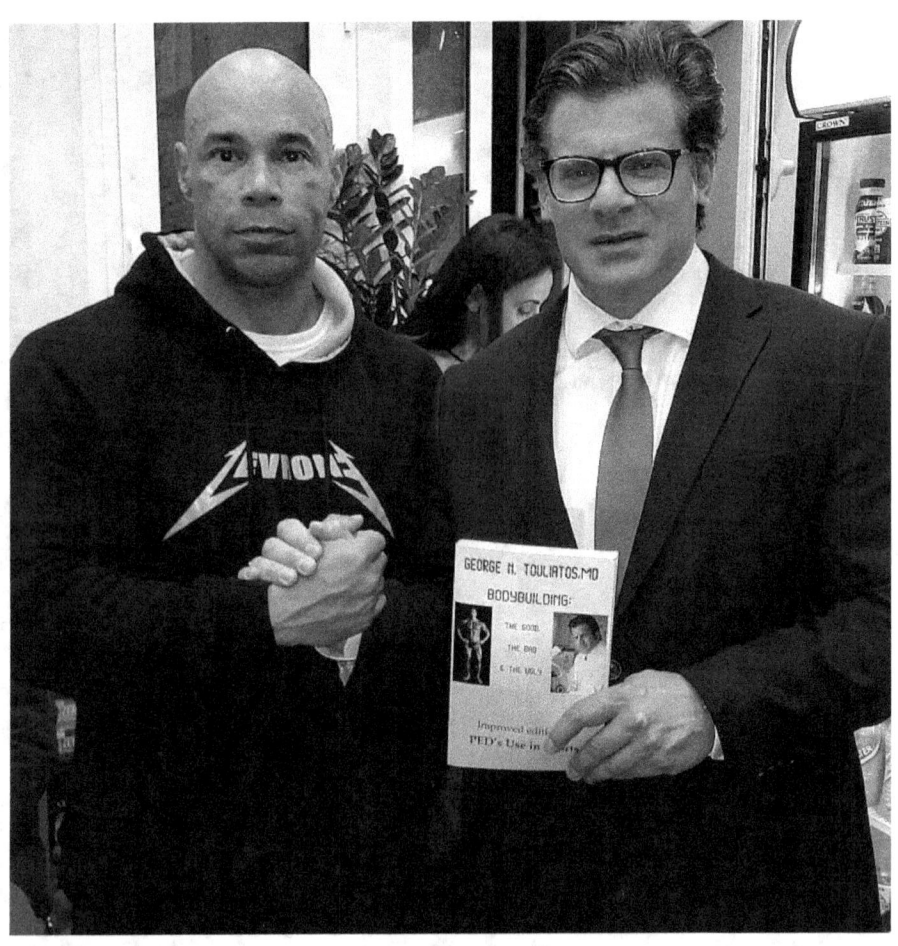

Kevin Levrone (USA)

ASC USA 1994,1996 champion

Mr.Olympia first runner up 1998

Owner of Kevin Levrone nutrition

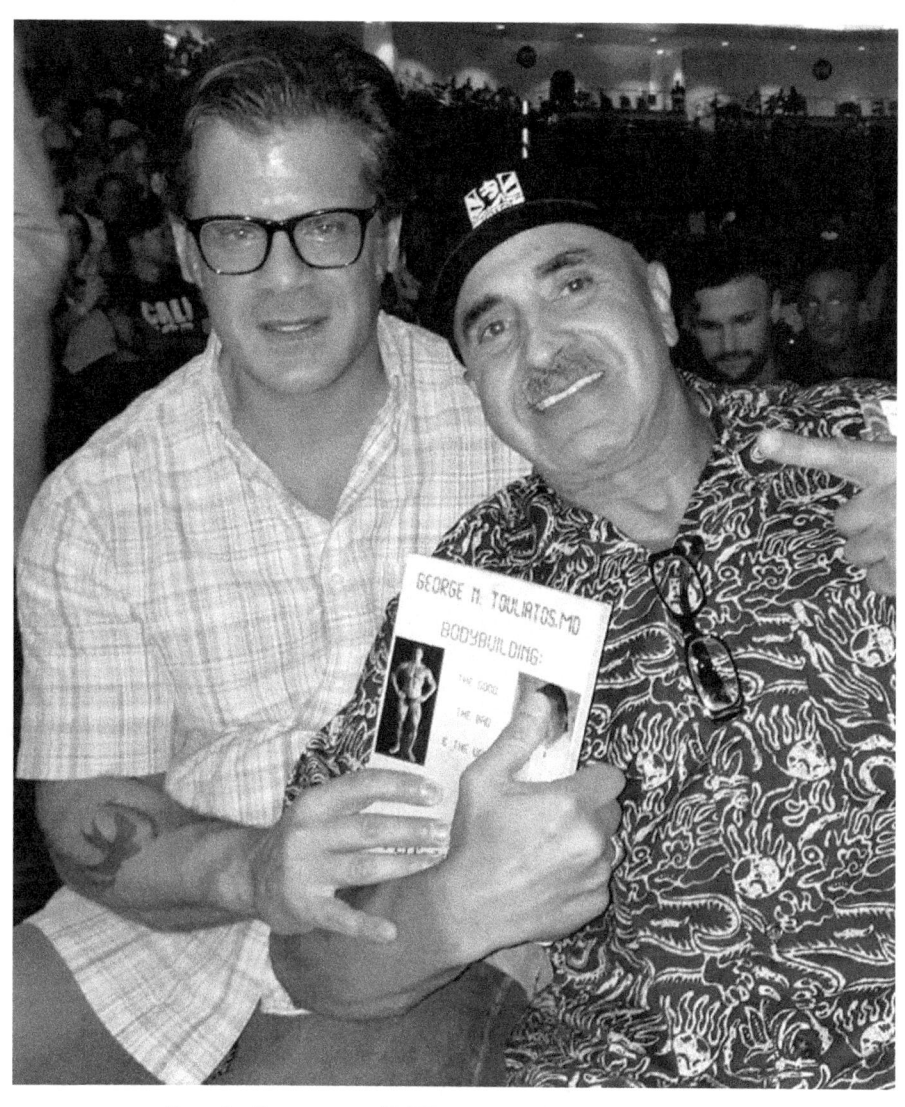

Samir Bannout (LEBANON) 1983 Mr.Olympia

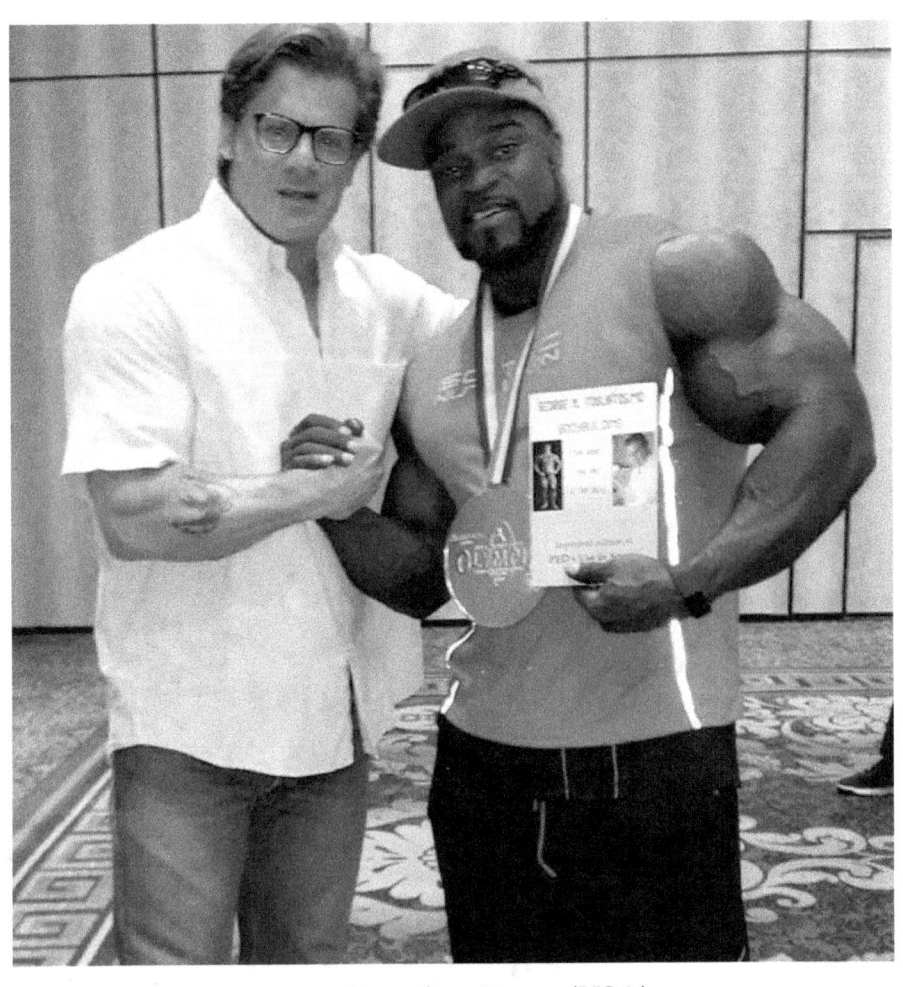

Brandon Curry (USA)

2019 ASC USA & Mr.Olympia champion

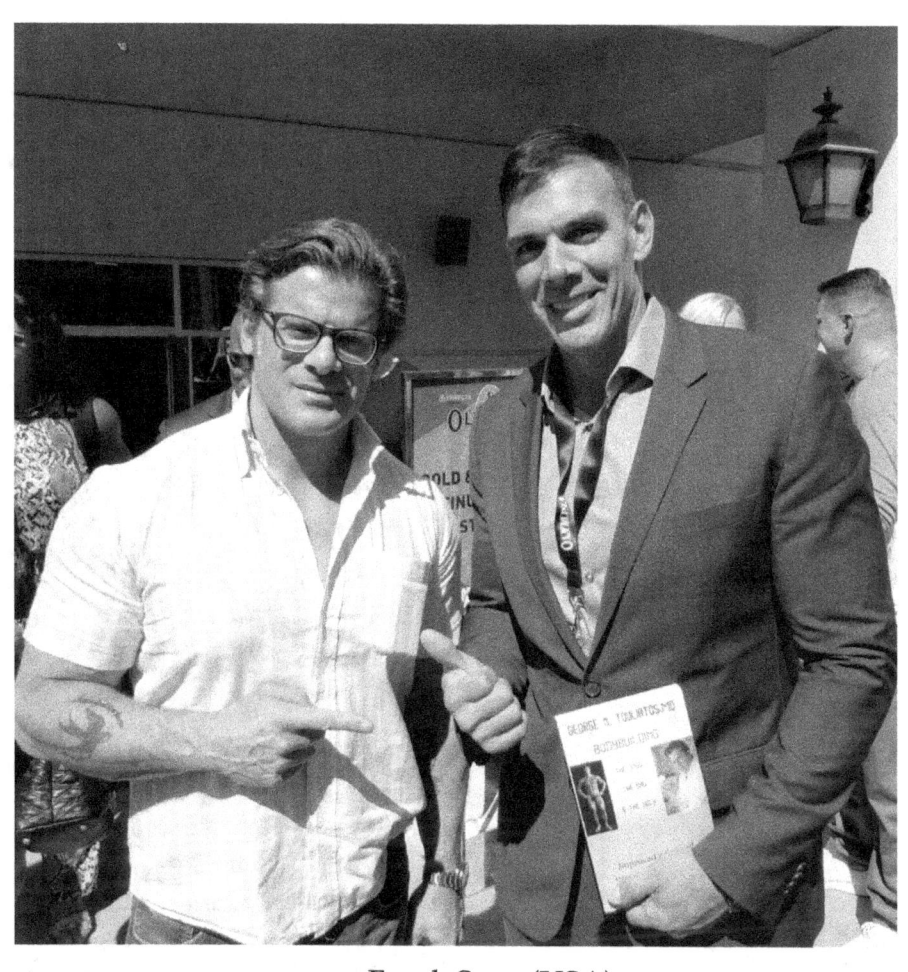

Frank Sepe (USA)

NPC News online chairman

Musclemag International columnist

Author in fitness, NPC superheavy weight competitor 1997

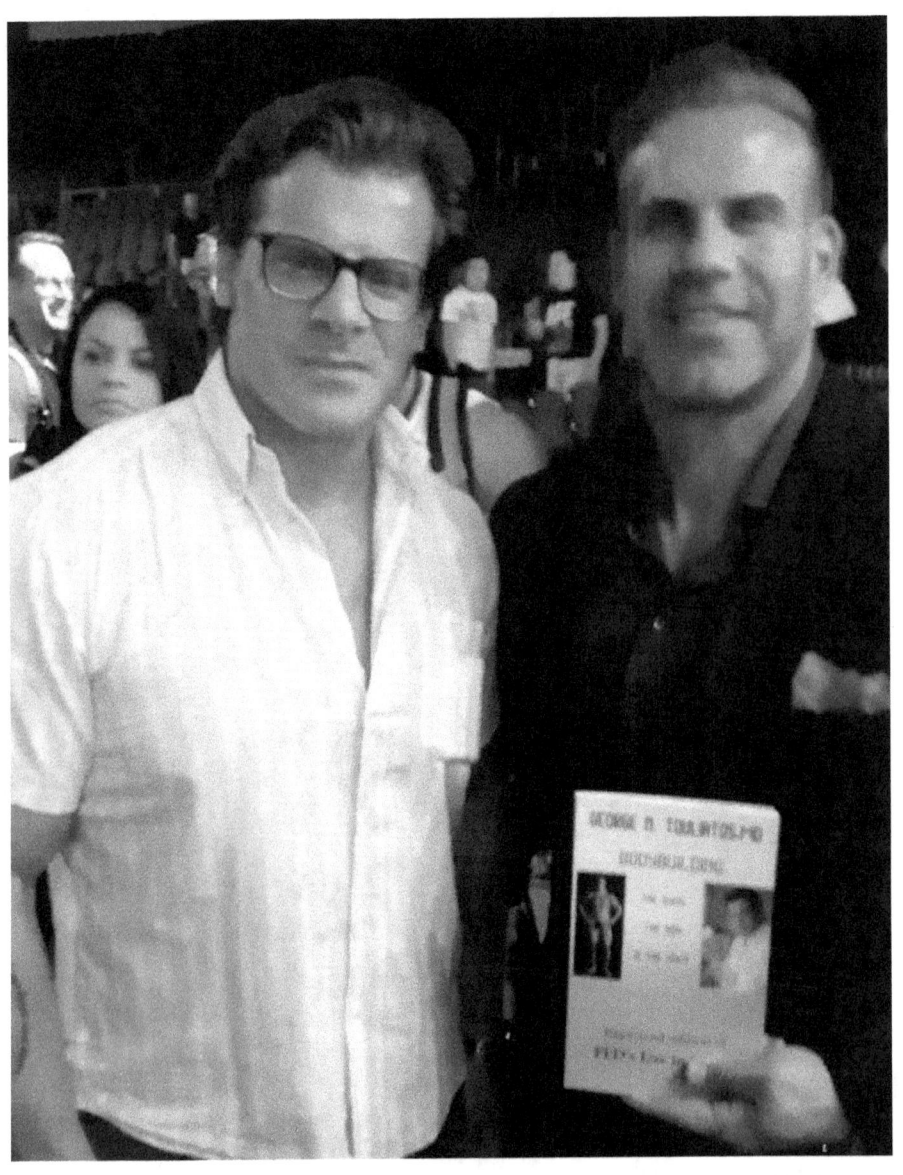

Jay Cutler (USA) Mr.Olympia 2006,2007,2009,2010
ASC USA 2002,2003,2004 champion
Owner of Cutler Nutrition

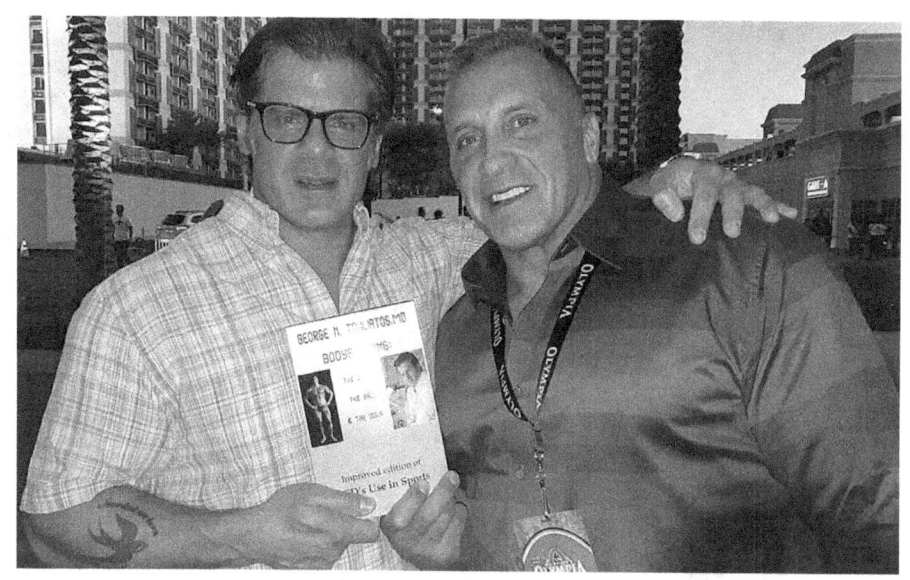

Milos Sarcev (SERBIA)
1997 Toronto Pro winner & Canada Pro winner

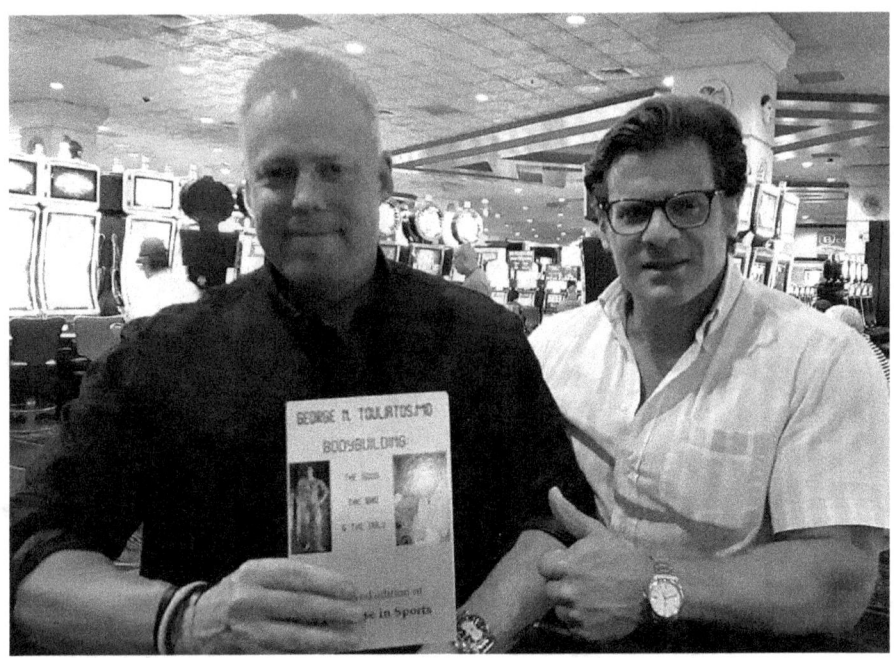

Rick Collins (USA) Attorney of the bodybuilding community, author of Legal Muscle, Collumnist of Muscular Development, competitive bodybuilder

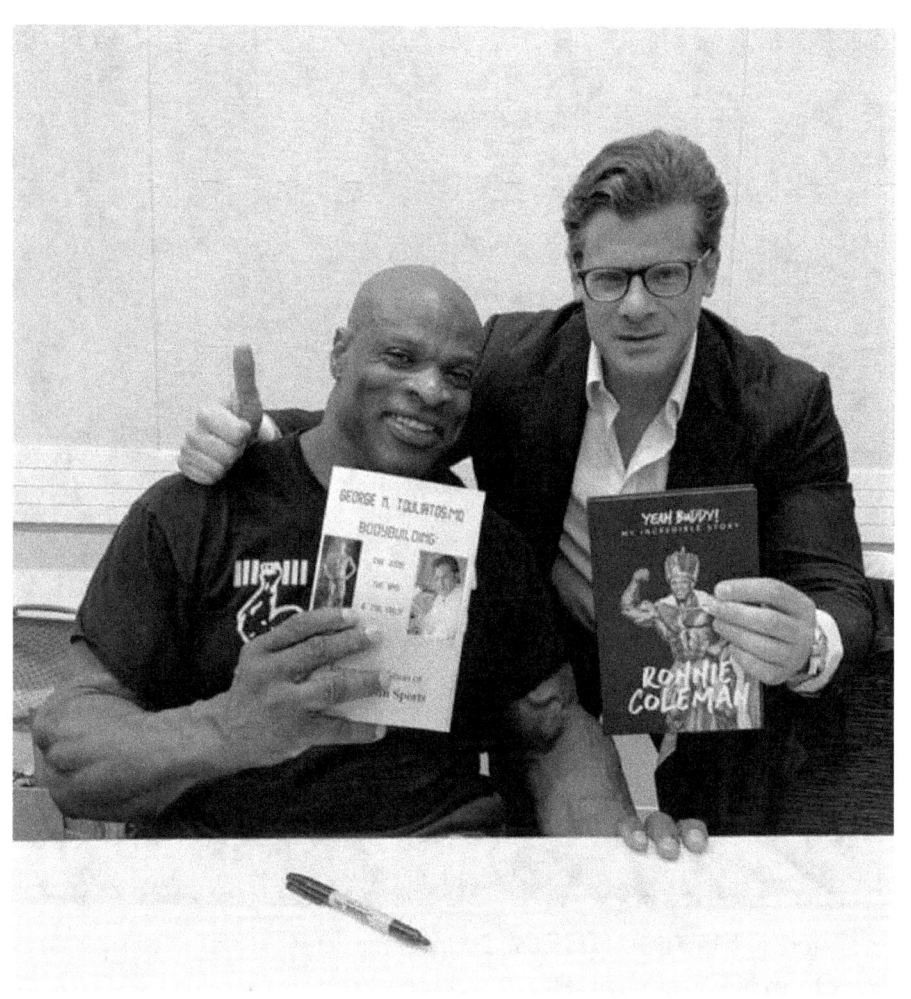

Ronnie Coleman (USA), 8x times Mr Olympia (1998-2005)

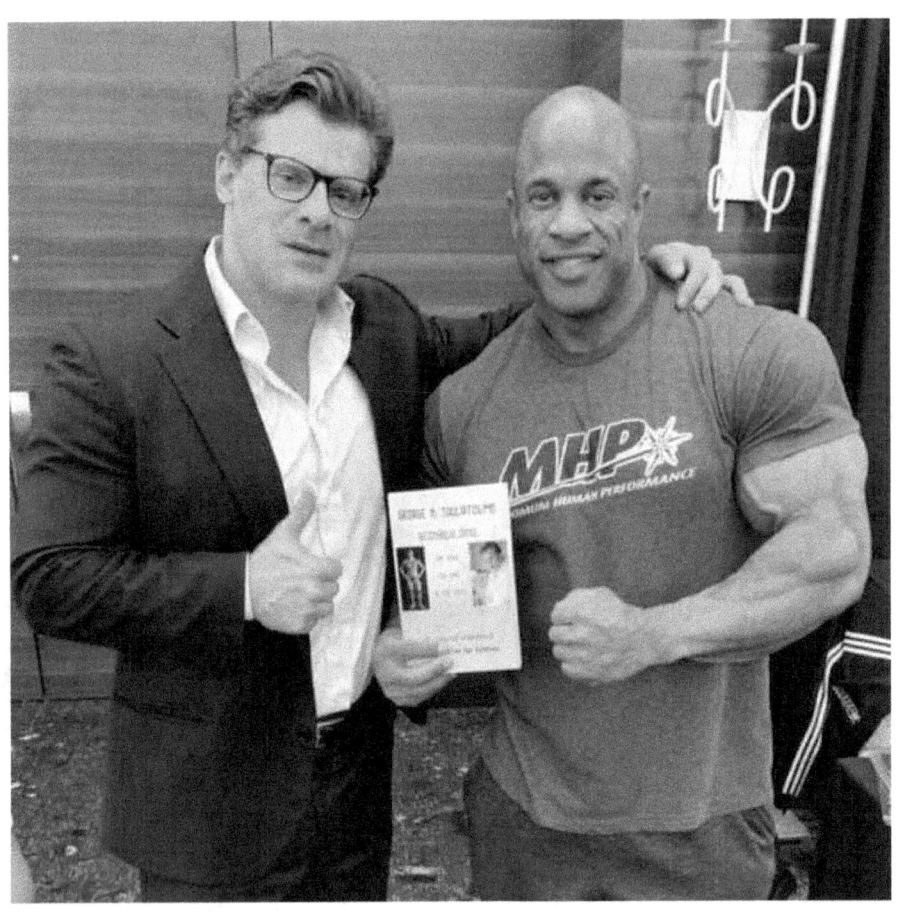

Victor Martinez (DRP) 2007 Arnold Classic champion & Mr.Olympia first runner up

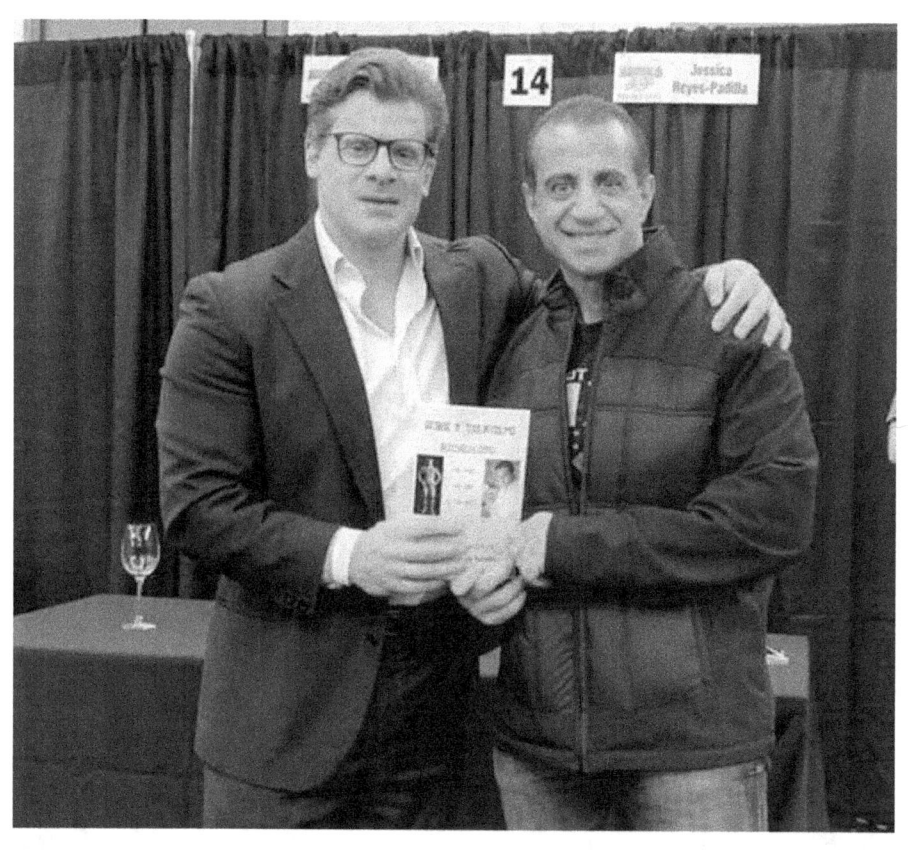

George Farah (LEBANON), Mr. Olympia competitor

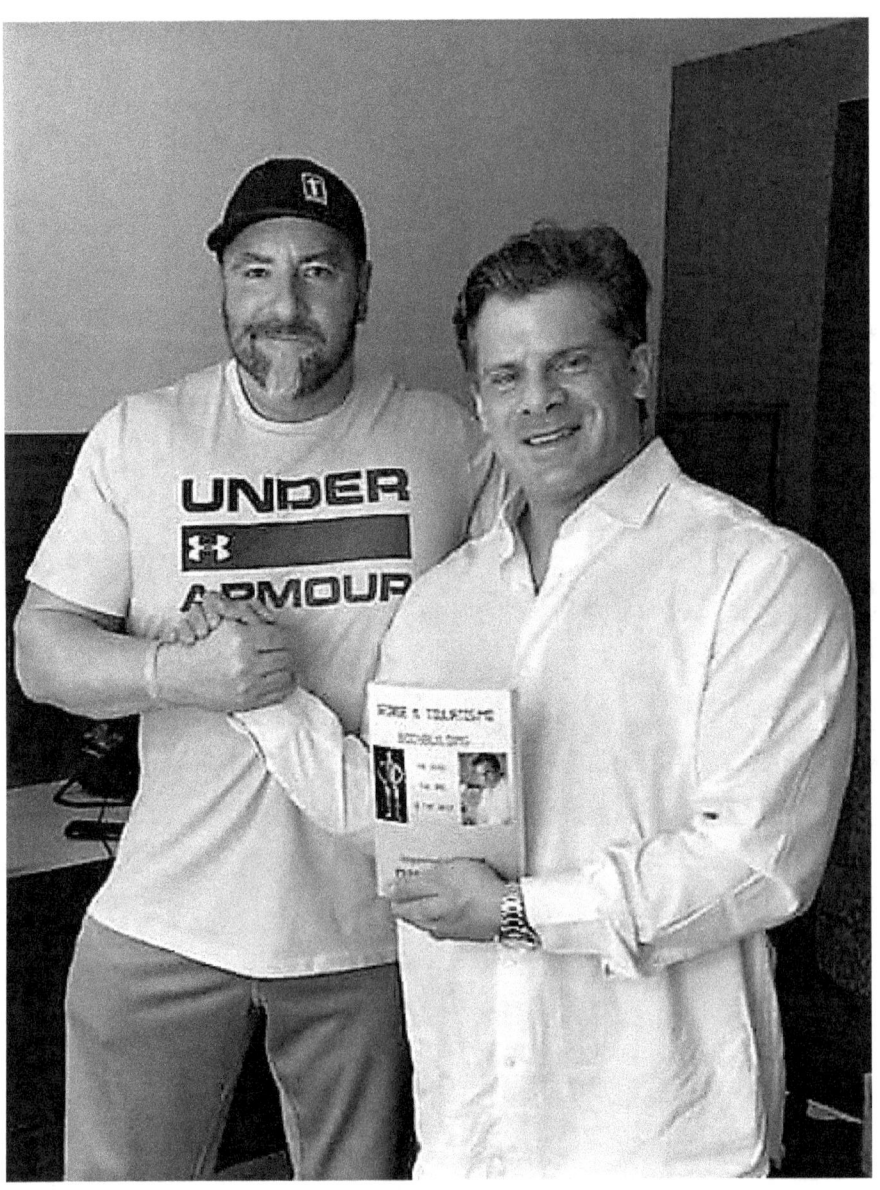

Chad Nickols (U.S.A) guru of Olympians

www.ingramcontent.com/pod-product-compliance
Lightning Source LLC
Chambersburg PA
CBHW052310220526
45472CB00001B/60

Find the e-Book on Amazon